Side-effects of Cancer Chemotherapy on the Gastrointestinal Tract

FALK WORKSHOP

Side-effects of Cancer Chemotherapy on the Gastrointestinal Tract

Pathophysiology, Prophylaxis and Therapy

Edited by

M. Staritz
Klinik für Innere Medizin I
Klinikum der Stadt Villingen-Schwenningen GmbH
Germany

G. Adler
Abteilung Innere Medizin I
Medizinische Universitätsklinik
Ulm
Germany

A. Knuth
Hämatologie/Onkologie
II. Medizinische Klinik
Krankenhaus Nordwest
Frankfurt, Germany

W. Schmiegel
Medizinische Universitätsklinik
Knappschaftskrankenhaus
Bochum-Langendreer
Germany

H.-J. Schmoll
Klinik und Poliklinik für Innere Medizin IV
Hämatologie/Onkologie
Martin-Luther-Universität Halle-Wittemberg
Halle, Germany

Proceedings of Falk Workshop held in Freiburg, Germany, October 11, 2002

KLUWER ACADEMIC PUBLISHERS
DORDRECHT / BOSTON / LONDON

Library of Congress Cataloging-in-Publication Data is available.

ISBN 0-7923-8791-0

Published by Kluwer Academic Publishers, BV
P.O. Box 17, 3300 AA Dordrecht, The Netherlands.

Sold and distributed in North, Central and South America
by Kluwer Academic Publishers,
101 Philip Drive, Norwell, MA 02061, USA.

In all other countries, sold and distributed
by Kluwer Academic Publishers, Distribution Center,
P.O. Box 322, 3300 AH Dordrecht, The Netherlands.

Printed on acid-free paper

Printed and bound in Great Britain by MPG Books, Bodmin, Cornwall.

Contents

* This contribution was not presented orally but included for completion of the section "Clinical Pharmacology".

Section III: SIDE-EFFECTS OF CHEMOTHERAPEUTIC AGENTS: PHYSIOLOGY, PATHOPHYSIOLOGY AND TERMINOLOGY

Section IV: ADVERSE EFFECTS OF CHEMOTHERAPEUTIC AGENTS – PATHOPHYSIOLOGY AND THERAPEUTIC APPROACHES

Section V: PERSPECTIVES, ALTERNATIVES

List of principal contributors

G Adler
Abteilung Innere Medizin I,
Medizinische Universitätsklinik Ulm
Robert-Koch-Str.1
D-89081 Ulm
Germany

MG Donelli
Dipartimento di Oncologia
Istituto di Ricerche
Farmacologiche Mario Negri
Via Eritrea 62
I-20157 Milano
Italy

M Fellhauer
Klinikum der Stadt Villingen-Schwenningen GmbH
Vöhrenbacher Str. 23
D-78050 Villingen-Schwenningen
Germany

W Fischbach
Medizinische Klinik II
Klinikum Aschaffenburg
Am Hasenkopf
D-63739 Aschaffenburg
Germany

PR Galle
I. Medizinische Klinik und Poliklinik
Johannes-Gutenberg-Universität Mainz
Langenbeckstr. 1
D-55131 Mainz
Germany

A Glasmacher
Medizinische Klinik und Poliklinik I
Allgemeine Innere Medizin
Universitätsklinikum Bonn
Sigmund-Freud-Str. 25
D-53105 Bonn
Germany

M Gorschlüter
Medizinische Klinik und Poliklinik I
Allgemeine Innere Medizin
Universitätsklinikum Bonn
Sigmund-Freud-Str. 25
D-53105 Bonn
Germany

JT Hartmann
Department of Hematology, Oncology, Immunology
UKT – Medical Center II
Eberhard-Karls-University Tübingen
Otfried-Müller-Str. 10
D-72076 Tübingen
Germany

D Jaeger
II. Medizinische Klinik
Krankenhaus Nordwest
Steinbacher Hohl 2-26
D-60488 Frankfurt
Germany

K Jordan
Innere Medizin IV
Martin-Luther-Universität
Halle-Wittenberg
Ernst-Grube-Str. 40
D-06120 Halle
Germany

W Kämmerer
Dr.-Horst-Schmidt-Kliniken GmbH
Ludiwg-Erhard-Str. 100
D-65199 Wiesbaden
Germany

A Knuth
Hämatologie/Onkologie
II. Medizinische Klinik
Krankenhaus Nordwest
Steinbacher Hohl 2-26
D-60488 Frankfurt
Germany

F Kullmann
Klinik für Innere Medizin I
Universität Regensburg
Franz-Josef-Strauß-Allee
D-93053 Regensburg
Germany

J Mössner
Universität Leipzig
Medizinische Klinik und Poliklinik II
Philipp-Rosenthal-Str. 27
D-04103 Leipzig
Germany

Y Nieto
University of Colorado
Bone Marrow Transplant Program
4200 East Ninth Avenue, B#190
Denver, Colorado 80262
USA

G Ramadori
Georg-August-Universität Göttingen
Abteilung Gastroenterologie und Endokrinologie
Robert-Koch-Str. 40
D-37075 Göttingen
Germany

A Rühl
Lehrstuhl für Humanbiologie
Technische Universität München
Hochfeldweg 2
D-85350 Freising-Weihenstephan
Germany

S Schmidt
Institut und Poliklinik für Medizinische Psychologie
Universitätsklinikum Hamburg
Martinistr. 52 Haus S35
D-20246 Hamburg
Germany

W Schmiegel
Medizinische Universitätsklinik
Knappschaftskrankenhaus Bochum-Langendreer
In der Schornau 23-25
D-44892 Bochum
Germany

H-J Schmoll
Klinik und Poliklinik für Innere Medizin IV
Hämatologie/Onkologie
Martin-Luther-Universität
Halle-Wittemberg
Ernst-Grube-Str. 40
D-06067 Halle
Germany

M Schultz
Klinik für Innere Medizin I
Universität Regensburg
Franz-Josef-Strauß-Allee
D-93053 Regensburg
Germany

J Siebler
I. Medizinische Klinik und
Poliklinik
Johannes-Gutenberg-Universität
Mainz
Langenbeckstr. 1
D-55131 Mainz
Germany

M Staritz
Klinik für Innere Medizin I – Gastroenterologie
Klinikum der Stadt Villingen-Schwenningen GmbH
Röntgenstr. 20
D-78054 Villingen-Schwenningen
Germany

Ch Wittekind
Institut für Pathologie
Universitätsklinikum Leipzig
Liebigstr. 26
D-04103 Leipzig
Germany

Preface 1

Cancer chemotherapy frequently attacks the gastrointestinal tract. Many of the possible side-effects reduce the patient's quality of life, may limit acceptance of further drug administration and even life-threatening complications must be considered. Contributions of pathologists, pharmacologists, oncologists and gastroenterologists should improve the understanding of the effects of anticancer agents on the organs of the gastrointestinal tract, and help to compensate for chemotherapy-induced adverse effects.

We are greatly indebted to the authors of the contributions and to Dr Herbert Falk and the Falk Foundation for generous support.

M Staritz

G Adler **A Knuth**

W Schmiegel **H-J Schmoll**

Preface 2

Chemotherapy in cancer patients is a complex treatment procedure, and has become more and more complicated with the advent of new anticancer drugs, multidrug combinations and targeted therapies. The interaction of the different agents, as well as the overlapping toxicities in multiple drug combinations, are sometimes difficult to understand, and require extensive clinical experience and consideration in an individual patient. The recent development of modern pharmacogenomics has provided an interesting insight into the individual reactions of a specific patient to the cytostatic agents; this might be even more important for antitumour activity than the cellular resistance level of the tumour cell itself. The different toxicities of the cytostatic agents limit the dose, the possibilities for combinations and therefore the antitumour activities. The molecular therapeutics raise further questions, since interactions with classical cytostatic agents are not yet known. Therefore, this entire workshop regarding the question of side-effects of cancer chemotherapy with particular reference to the gastrointestinal tract is of great importance. It is also very important that this symposium has an interdisciplinary orientation, since several disciplines are now participating in the treatment of patients with cancer. It is very much appreciated that the chairman of this symposium, Professor Staritz, has chosen a group of colleagues from different societies and fields to prepare this interesting symposium.

H-J Schmoll

Section I
Clinical pharmacology of cancer chemotherapy drugs

1
Pharmacology of cancer chemotherapy drugs

M. STARITZ and M. FELLHAUER

INTRODUCTION

Most of the agents available for cancer chemotherapy (Table 1) inhibit nucleic acid synthesis or function during replication or transcription (Figure 1). Nucleic acid synthesis is a complex process which needs several participants. These participants are:

1. Substrates (dATP, dCTP, dGTP, dTTP). Substrate comprises agents that interfere with the synthesis of purine and pyrimidine bases and therefore ultimately interfere with nucleic acid synthesis.
2. DNA template (native double-stranded DNA). Disruption of the template causes disruption of nucleic acid synthesis.
3. Enzymes (polymerases, nucleases, ligases and topoisomerases I and II). Inhibition of these enzymes causes inhibition of nucleic acid synthesis.

The site of action of different anticancer drugs is outlined in Figure 1.

DRUGS AND PRODRUGS

Most of the anticancer chemotherapy drugs present as directly acting agents. Some of the most frequently used drugs, however, are prodrugs which need activation in the liver or even in the individual tumour cells (Table 2). The site of activation and the mechanism of activation are outlined in Table 3 and are subjects of further investigation. Sometimes the mechanism of activation is speculative and has not really been scientifically elucidated.

Table 1 Cancer chemotherapy drugs (selection)

Mechanism of action	*International non-proprietary name (INN)*
Alkylating agents	Cyclophosphamide, cisplatin, oxaliplatin
Antimetabolites	Methotrexate, 5-fluorouracil (5-FU), cytarabine, 6-mercaptopurine, fludarabine phosphate
Cytostatic antibiotics	Dactinomycin (actinomycin D), bleomycin, daunomycin and doxorubicin
Antimitotic agents	Vinca alkaloids (vinblastine, vincristine); taxol (Paclitaxel)
Topoisomerase I inhibitors	Irinotecan (CPT-11)
Hormones and hormone-related agents	Antioestrogen (tamoxifen), antiandrogen (flutamide)

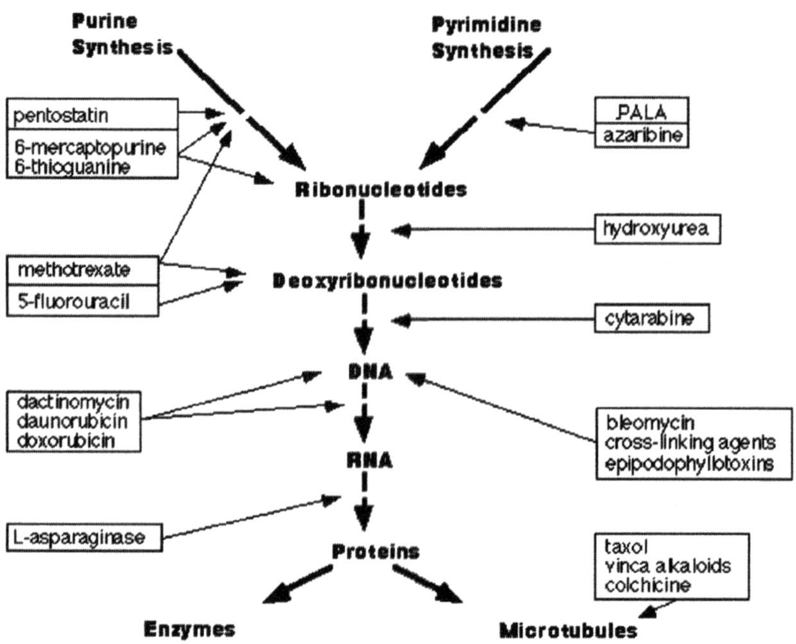

Figure 1 Site of action of various anticancer drugs

PHARMACOKINETIC VARIABILITY

Anticancer chemotherapy drugs may show a considerable variability in the individual patient. There are factors improving efficacy and factors diminishing anticancer potency. Individual conditions which may decrease absorption in the small bowel are nausea and vomiting, or surgery affecting the gastrointestinal unit. The effect of radiation on the small bowel should also be considered. In lipophilic drugs the effect of dereased body fat may be important in patients who

Table 2 Mechanism of action of anticancer agents

Mechanism of action	*INN*	*Prodrug*
Alkylating agents	Cyclophosphamide	Yes
	Cisplatin	—
	Carboplatin	—
Antimetabolites	Methotrexate	—
	Gemcitabine	—
	Capecitabine	Yes
	Fluorouracil	—
Cytostatic antibiotics	Doxorubicin	—
	Epirubicin	—
Antimitotic agents	Paclitaxel	—
	Etoposide	—
	Vincristine	—
Topoisomerase I inhibitors	Irinotecan	Yes
	Topotecan	-

Table 3 Prodrugs, site and mechanism of activation

INN	*Site of activation*	*Mechanism of activation*
Cyclophosphamide	Hepatic and intracellular	Enzymatic transformation to active alkylating metabolites acrolein and phosphoramide mustard
Capecitabine	Selectively tumour-activated	Transformation to its active metabolite fluorouracil, thymidine phosphorylase
Irinotecan	Primarily hepatic	Rapidly converted to its active metabolite SN-38, by hepatic carboxylesterase enzymes

Table 4 Aetiologic factors influencing pharmacokinetic variability of cytostatics

Absorption (oral drugs)	↓	Nausea/vomiting
	↓	Surgery affecting gastrointestinal tract
	↓	Radiation
	↓↑	Drug–drug interaction
Distribution	↓	Body weight loss
	↓	Decreased body fat (lipophilic drugs)
	↑	Hypoalbuminaemia
Metabolism	↓	Hepatic dysfunction
Elimination	↓	Renal dysfunction
	↓	Hepatic dysfunction

have lost body weight (Table 4). Most of the drugs are transported by albumin; thus hypoalbuminaemia may play an important and not clearly elucidated role. Since clearance of drugs is provided by liver and kidneys the effect of impaired function of liver and kidney should be mentioned. Only a few clinical studies are available to define the effect of impaired function of liver and kidney and pharmacokinetic availability of anticancer chemotherapy drugs. Finally the clinical relevance of drug–drug interaction has not been investigated.

PHARMACOKINETIC PARAMETERS OF ANTICANCER CHEMOTHERAPY DRUGS

Pharmacokinetic parameters of anticancer agents are not yet clearly identified; nevertheless a large variability of terminal half-life could be identified. Particularly a large interindividual variety of half-life (cisplatin 2–96 h) may explain unexpected severe side-effects in individual patients. Since the main route of excretion is, in most of the agents, provided by the kidney and/or the liver – a wide range of pharmacokinetic characteristics may be presented, particularly in patients with impaired function of liver and/or kidney (Table 5).

CHARACTERISTICS OF CANCER CHEMOTHERAPY DRUGS

Alkylating agents

Cyclophosphamide

Cyclophosphamide is an alkylating agent derived from nitrogen mustard. Its mother compound, "Lost", was used during World War I; victims showed aplasia of bone marrow and dissolution of lymphoid tissue. The chemical structure shows a biofunctional alkylating group. The mechanism of action of alkylating agents comprises modification of nucleic acids and a nucleophilic attack of the purine ring. It causes inter-strand crosslinks and disrupts DNA synthesis. The drug is activated by the hepatic cytochrome P450 system.

Table 5 Pharmacokinetic characteristics

Mechanism of action	*INN*	*Terminal half-life*	*Metabolism*	*Excretion (main route)*
Alkylating agents	Cyclophosphamide	4–10 h	Yes	Renal
	Cisplatin	2–96 h	Yes	Renal
	Carboplatin	6 h	(Yes)	Renal
Antimetabolites	Methotrexate	8–15 h	Yes	Renal
	Gemcitabine	0.7–1.6 h	Yes	Renal
	Capecitabine	0.75 h	Yes	Renal
	Fluorouracil	0.2–0.3 h	Yes	Renal
Cytostatic antibiotics	Doxorubicin	29 h	Yes	Biliary
	Epirubicin	30–40 h	Yes	Biliary
Antimitotic agents	Paclitaxel	6–13 h	Yes	Biliary
	Etoposide	4–11 h	Yes	Renal
	Vincristine	85 h	Yes	Biliary
Topoisomerase I inhibitors	Irinotecan	11.7 h	Yes	Biliary/renal
	Topotecan	2–3 h	Yes	Biliary/renal

Pharmacokinetics
Cyclophosphamide is well absorbed orally. Upon activation in the liver it is transported to the target site by the circulatory system. Variability of antitumour activity is based on patient variability in activating enzyme levels.

Resistance
Resistance occurs commonly. Well-established reasons are

1. Decreased permeability for activated drug.
2. Increased production of glutathione, which can compete with target DNA for alkylation.
3. An increase in DNA repair enzyme levels.
4. Increased metabolism of activated drug to inactive forms by aldehyde dehydrogenase.

Adverse effects
Most common severe adverse effects are acute myelosuppression (nadir within a week, recovery within 3 weeks) and suppression of cellular and humoral immunities. Acrolein, a metabolite of cyclophosphamide, is nephrotoxic; the substance can cause pulmonary fibrosis, nausea and vomiting.

Clinical applications
Administered orally or intravenously. The drug is used extensively in the treatment of non-Hodgkin's lymphoma, Burkitt's lymphoma and as and adjuvant therapy following surgery for breast carcinoma.

Cisplatin

Cisplatin is a divalent inorganic, water-soluble platinum-containing complex. The drug reacts directly with DNA, resulting in both intra- and interstrand crosslinks. It inhibits DNA replication and RNA transcription, and leads to DNA breaks.

Pharmacokinetics
Cisplatin is administered intravenously, the plasma half-life is greater than 50 min and more than 90% is bound by plasma proteins. High concentrations are found in the kidney, liver, intestine and testes. It is excreted by the kidneys.

Resistance
Increased levels of DNA-excision repair enzymes.

Adverse effects
Adverse effects comprise nephrotoxicity and ototoxicity. Many patients complain of nausea and vomiting, mild-to-moderate myelosuppression and anaphylactic-like reactions.

Clinical applications
The drug is highly successful in combination therapies with other anticancer drugs in the treatment of testicular and ovarian cancers, also cancers of the

bladder, head, neck, and endometrium. It sensitizes cells to the cytotoxic effects of radiation therapy.

Oxaliplatin

Oxaliplatin is a cytotoxic alkylating agent. As a third-generation platinum compound it is considered to be more cytotoxic than cisplatin and carboplatin, but the exact mechanism of action is not known. It differs from cisplatin and carboplatin in having a broader spectrum of antitumour activity. Molecular studies suggest that oxaliplatin adducts are recognized and processed in a different way compared to those produced by the earlier-generation platinum-containing drugs. Oxaliplatin is not generally cross-resistant to cisplatin or carboplatin, and the action is not cell cycle-specific.

Pharmacokinetics
Oxaliplatin is administered intravenously and metabolized by non-enzymatic transformation to platin complexes. Excretion is primarily renal with a terminal half-life (platinum) of 273 h.

Resistance
It has been shown that the development of acquired resistance to oxaliplatin is accompanied by defects in cell uptake and in DNA adduct formation.

Adverse effects
The emetogenic potential is moderate to high. Nausea and vomiting occur in 70%. Peripheral sensory neuropathy may be dose-limiting. This side-effect is dose-related and usually reversible after a few months. Elderly patients are at higher risk for severe diarrhoea. Incidences of adverse effects are similar with oxaliplatin as single agent or with a 5-FU and leucovorin combination, but there is more severe diarrhoea, nausea and vomiting and neurotoxicity with combination therapy.

Clinical application
Oxaliplatin is primarily used in colorectal cancer; other uses are breast, gastric, germ cell, head and neck, lung cancer and non-Hodgkin's lymphoma.

Antimetabolites

Methotrexate (Figure 2)

Methotrexate has been used since 1948 when the first temporary remission of leukaemia was achieved. Methotrexate is a folic acid analogue (single carbon donor in biosynthetic pathways); its mechanism of action is characterized by inhibition of dihydrofolate reductase.

Pharmacokinetics
Low doses are applied orally, high doses must be administered intravenously. Renal clearance ($t_{1/2}$ = 2–3 h). Toxic effects increase with impaired renal function. Can be sequestered in ascites fluid, act as storage (prolonged high plasma concentrations). Only 3% in cerebrospinal fluid, only effective against central nervous system tumours at high doses.

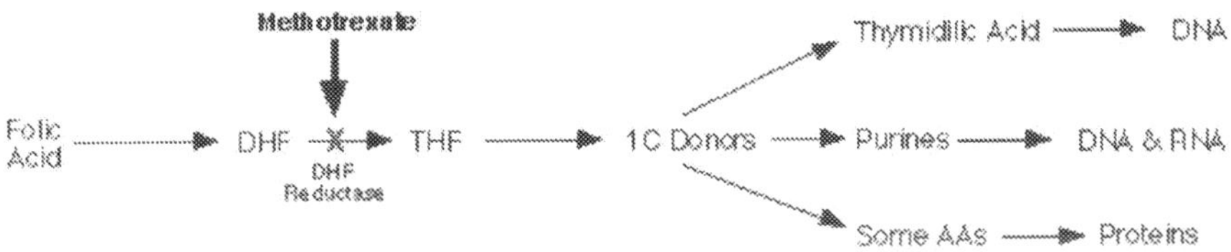

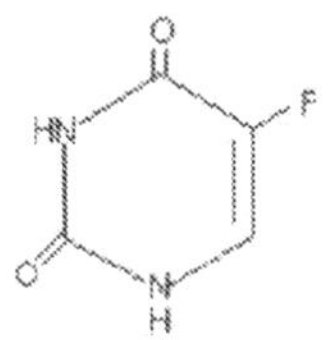

5-FLUOROURACIL

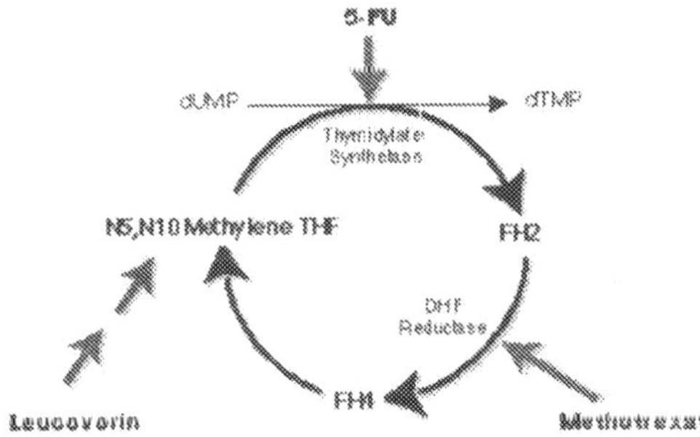

Resistance
Resistance is developed by decreased transport into cells, decreased affinity of dihydrafolate (DHF) reductase for methotrexate and increased levels of DHF reductase by gene amplification and/or loss of autoregulatory control of expression.

Adverse effects
The most common adverse effects are inflammation of intestinal epithelium, bone marrow suppression, mucositis, alopecia and nephrotoxicity.

Clinical applications

1. Childhood acute lymphoblastic leukaemia.
2. Choriocarcinoma.
3. Osteosarcoma.
4. Non-Hodgkin's and Burkitt's lymphoma.

5-Fluorouracil (5-FU)

The chemical structure is a halogenated pyrimidine ring. 5-FU binding is stronger than the normal C–H bond which prevents thymidylate synthetase from methylating the ring. It also inhibits RNA processing and is, erroneously, incorporated into DNA. 5-FU is activated by conversion to the nucleotide (ribosylation and phosphorylation).

Pharmacokinetics
5-FU is normally administered parenterally. Inactivation is caused by reduction of the pyrimidine ring by dihydropyrimidine dehydrogenase. Patients who are

deficient in this activity develop increased sensitivity to 5-FU. Elimination half-life of the parent compound is 6–22 minutes; about 10–20% are excreted renally.

Resistance
Tumour cells develop resistance by decreased levels of activating enzymes, amplification of thymidylate synthetase and/or loss of autoregulatory control of expression.

Adverse effects
Adverse effects appear delayed. Most common are anorexia, nausea, stomatitis and diarrhoea. Myelosuppression occurs 9–14 days after the first injection. Alopecia, acute cerebellar syndrome and cardiac toxicity may appear delayed. Close supervision of 5-FU administration is necessary due to various and severe toxicities.

Clinical applications
5-FU is used for therapy of metastatic breast carcinomas; also ovarian, prostate, pancreatic and hepatic carcinomas. It is an effective drug for adjuvant and palliative treatment of colorectal carcinoma.

Cytarabine

Cytarabine is a structure–analogue of 2-deoxycytidine; its mechanism of action is provided by a stereoisomer of deoxycytidine (3-OH *trans*, not *cis* configuration) that results in steric hindrance of pyrimidine base rotation around the nucleosidic bond. It causes impaired base stacking when incorporated into the DNA helix. Cytarabine must be activated to AraCMP by deoxycytidine kinase. AraCTP inhibits DNA synthesis at the elongation step, leading to chain termination.

Pharmacokinetics
Oral administration results in 20% absorption (degraded in the gastrointestinal tract). Initial and terminal half-lives are 10 minutes and 2 hours, respectively. Half-life in cerebrospinal fluid is approximately 2 h.

Resistance
Resistance is caused by a deficiency in deoxycytidine kinase, expansion of the deoxycytidine triphosphate (dCTP) pool by increased dCTP synthase activity.

Adverse effects
Most common adverse effects are myelosuppression, gastrointestinal disturbances and reversible hepatic dysfunction. Neurotoxicity may occur when the drug is administered in high doses.

Clinical applications
Cytarabine is the most effective agent in inducing the remission of acute myelocytic leukaemia.

6-Mercaptopurine

The structure of 6-mercaptopurine is a thio-substituted purine ring, analogue to hypoxanthine and guanine. It is a prodrug which must be activated to the nucleotide to be cytotoxic. It is an excellent substrate for hypoxanthine–guanine phosphoribosyltransferase (HGPRT). It leads to the accumulation of 6-thioinosine-5-phosphate (T-IMP), which inhibits enzymes critical to purine nucleotide synthesis. Metabolites also act as pseudofeedback regulators of purine synthesis.

Pharmacokinetics
Oral administration and first-pass metabolism by liver results in 5–37% bioavailability. Plasma levels must be monitored to optimize therapy.

Resistance
Resistance occurs by decreased transport, decreased HGPRT levels, decreased affinity for HGPRT, increased degradation by xanthine oxidase (co-administer allopurinol to inhibit xanthine oxidase). Cross-resistance does not occur between mercaptopurine and other classes of antileukaemic drugs.

Adverse effects
Most common adverse effects are bone marrow depression, anorexia, nausea and vomiting. Sometimes jaundice occurs associated with hepatic necrosis.

Clinical applications
The drug is used for therapy of acute lymphoblastic leukaemia (maintenance of remissions) and chronic granulocytic leukaemia.

Fludarabine phosphate

The chemical structure shows a fluorinated nucleotide analogue of vidarabine (antiviral agent). The substance is rapidly dephosphorylated at the membrane and rephosphorylated intracellularly by deoxycytidine kinase to the active triphosphate derivative. It inhibits DNA polymerase and DNA primase. The substance is incorporated into DNA and RNA. The full mechanism of cytotoxicity is not yet completely understood.

Pharmacokinetics
The drug is administered intravenously by infusion over 30–120 min. Terminal half-life is 10 h. It is eliminated by renal excretion.

Resistance
The development of resistance is not yet well characterized.

Adverse effects
The most common adverse effects are myelosuppression, nausea, vomiting, chills and fever. $CD4^+$ cells are depleted and opportunistic infections may occur. Caution is required in patients with impaired renal function.

Clinical applications
The agent is used for therapy of chronic lymphocytic leukaemia and low-grade lymphomas.

Cytostatic antibiotics

Dactinomycin (actinomycin D)

Dactinomycin has been isolated from *Streptomyces* species. The molecular strucure shows a chromopeptide (highly coloured), containing a planar chromophore with peptide side-chains. The drug causes intercalation in the minor groove of double-stranded DNA and interferes with RNA polymerase and with topoisomerase II.

Pharmacokinetics
Oral administration is possible but with insufficient resorption. Parenteral administration is preferred. The drug is excreted in bile and urine; the half-life is 36 h.

Resistance
The basis of drug resistance of cancer cells is not yet elucidated.

Adverse effects
Adverse effects are anorexia, nausea, vomiting (immediate), bone marrow suppression and alopecia (subsequently). A severe local toxicity as a result of inadvertent extravasation during administration should be mentioned.

Clinical applications
Curative in combination with surgery, radiotherapy, and other drugs in treating rhabdomyosarcoma and Wilm's tumour in children.

Bleomycin

Bleomycin is a naturally occurring fermentation product of *Streptomyces verticillus*. Its structure shows an A basic glycoprotein, which is complexed with the metal cations Cu^{2+} and Fe^{2+}.

Mechanism of action
The drug causes fragmentation of DNA and separates electrons from complexed metal cations which are transferred to molecular O_2. DNA is attacked by superoxide and –OH radicals.

Pharmacokinetics
The substance must be administered parenterally. It can be instilled locally to treat bladder cancer. The half-time for elimination is approximately 3 h. It is primarily excreted in the urine. A reduced dosage is recommended in patients with impaired renal function.

Resistance
Resistance of cancer cells may be caused by increased hydrolase activity and increased DNA repair activity.

Adverse effects
Adverse effects are significant cutaneous and pulmonary toxicity due to low hydrolase activity in the skin and lungs. Pulmonary toxicity may progress to life-threatening pulmonary fibrosis. Hyperthermia, headache, nausea and vomiting are common. Minimal myelosuppression should be taken into account.

Clinical applications
The drug is highly effective in treating testicular and ovarian cancers. It is also successful for treatment of lymphomas in combination with other drugs.

Daunomycin and doxorubicin

Daunomycin and doxorubicin are derived from *Streptomyces*. The chemical structure shows a tetracyclic ring structure.

Mechanism of action
Daunomycin and doxorubicin cause intercalation of DNA, causing inhibition of DNA and RNA synthesis. The drugs lead to double-strand breaks, mediated either by topoisomerase II or the generation of free radicals.

Pharmacokinetics
Both drugs are administered intravenously. A rapid clearance from the plasma has been shown. Due to multiphasic elimination, half-lives between 3 and 30 h are possible. Metabolites are eliminated by conversion to inactive products.

Resistance
Resistance may be developed by increased glutathione peroxidase activity and decreased topoisomerase II activity.

Adverse effects
Major adverse effects are myelosuppression, alopecia and gastrointestinal disturbances. Most important is a cardiac toxicity that is dose-related and cumulative. This side-effect is manifested by congestive heart failure which is unresponsive to digitalis (> 50% fatal). The limit cumulative dose is 550 mg/m^2. Significant cardiomyopathies occur in more than 10% of patients, particularly in cumulative doses of more than 450 mg/m^2.

Clinical applications
Daunorubicin is effective in the treatment of acute lymphocytic and acute granulocytic leukaemias. It is most effective in the treatment of acute non-lymphoblastic leukaemias. Doxorubicin is used for the treatment of acute leukaemias, malignant lymphomas and solid tumours of the breast.

Antimitotic agents

Vinca alkaloids (vinblastine, vincristine)

The action of these drugs is cell-cycle-specific, blocking cells in M phase. They bind specifically to tubulin (molar ratio 1:1), inhibiting the polymerization of microtubules, leading to apoptotic signals and programmed cell death for both normal and malignant cells.

Pharmacokinetics
Vinca alkaloids are administered intravenously, metabolized by the liver and excreted in the bile. The half-life is approximately 20 h.

Resistance
Resistance is caused by the multidrug resistance efflux pump. Sometimes tubulin molecules are altered, causing reduced affinity for vinca alkaloids.

Adverse effects
Vincristine shows limited myelosuppression, but cumulative neutrotoxicity. It causes severe constipation at high doses. Vinblastine additionally causes myelosuppression. Gastrointestinal disturbances occur very often. Extravasation of drug during injection leads to cellulitis and phlebitis.

Clinical applications
Vincristine is very successful in the treatment of childhood leukaemias, Hodgkin's and non-Hodgkin's lymphoma, testicular and ovarian carcinomas, brain tumours and neuroblastoma.

Vinblastine offers curative therapy of metastatic testicular cancer. It is also effective in treating lymphomas, Kaposi's sarcoma and neuroblastoma.

Taxol (paclitaxel)

Taxanes have been isolated from the bark of the Western yew tree. The substance is now commercially semisynthesized from yew tree leaves. The molecular structure shows a diterpinoid compound with a complex taxane ring. Further modifications have led to the more potent analogue docetaxel. Paclitaxel promotes the polymerization of microtubules and binds specifically to b-tubulin.

Pharmacokinetics
Taxol is not water-soluble; the solubility is limited to 50% ethanol/50% polyethoxylated castor oil. Patients must be protected with corticosteroids and both H_1 and H_2 antihistamine prior to administration, generally in a 3–24 h infusion. The drug is primarily metabolized by the liver (P-450 system). Less than 10% is excreted in the urine intact.

Resistance
The basis of clinical drug resistance is not known.

Adverse effects
Taxol produces bone marrow suppression and severe peripheral neuropathy.

Clinical applications
Taxol is very effective in the treatment of metastatic ovarian and breast cancer. Early trials indicate significant response in cancer of the lung, head, neck, oesophageal and bladder carcinomas.

Topoisomerase I (Topo I) inhibitors

Irinotecan (CPT-11)

Irinotecan, a topoisomerase I inhibitor, is a derivative of camptothecin, a cytotoxic alkaloid from the Chinese tree *Camptotheca acuminata* (Xi Shu). The compound and its active metabolite SN-38 bind to the Topo I–DNA complex, resulting in double-strand DNA breakage and cell death. The cytotoxic action is cell cycle-specific.

Pharmacokinetics
Irinotecan is administered intravenously. Metabolism is primarily hepatic, by conversion to SN-38, the active metabolite. Terminal half-life is 12 h (irinotecan) and 21 h (SN-38). There is no clinically significant difference in pharmacokinetic parameters according to gender or age. Excretion is primarily via faeces (64%).

Resistance
Several mechanisms are discussed as possible causes for drug resistance of camptothecins: (a) variable levels of the enzymes involved in the conversion of irinotecan; (b) reduced cellular accumulation from active drug efflux; (c) reduced levels of Topo I expression; (d) alterations in the structure of Topo I from different mutations; (e) alterations in the cellular response to camptothecin–Topo I–DNA complex formation, which involves proteasome degradation of Topo I and/or enhanced DNA repair; and (f) activation of the transcription factor nuclear factor kappa B by DNA damage and subsequent suppression of apoptosis (from Xu Y. et al., 2002).

Adverse effects
The most common and dose-limiting side-effects are neutropenia and diarrhoea. Early-onset diarrhoea occurs within the first 24 h of administration, late-onset diarrhoea occurs more than 24 h after administration and may lead to life-threatening dehydration and electrolyte imbalance. The median duration is 3 days; severe diarrhoea should be treated with high-dose loperamide. Neutropenia may be increased in patients with hyperbilirubinaemia. The emetogenic potential is moderate–high, and there is no potential for extravasation hazard.

Clinical application
Irinotecan is used for colorectal cancer, and is being studied in several other tumour conditions.

Hormones and hormone-related agents

Tumours derived from hormone-sensitive tissues may be hormone-dependent. Once this property has been objectivated their growth can be inhibited by hormones with opposing actions, by hormone antagonists, or by agents that inhibit the synthesis of the stimulatory hormone.

Mechanism of action
Steroid hormones diffuse across the cell membrane, bind to a specific receptor, then this whole complex crosses the nuclear membrane and binds to a genomic

receptor. This action influences transcription and promotes proliferation of steroid-dependent tumours; therefore treatment could consist of removing the source of the influencing steroids. A common example is surgical gland removal in prostate cancer. Another mechanism of action is inhibiting the synthesis and/or binding of the influencing steroid.

Antioestrogen (tamoxifen)

Mechanism of action
Tamoxifen is a competitive inhibitor of oestradiol binding to the oestrogen receptor. The tamoxifen–receptor complex does not bind to the oestrogen response element, which normally initiates the expression of factors (TGF-β, IGF-1) that promote the growth of breast cancer cells.

Pharmacokinetics
Tamoxifen is administered orally. Metabolic products retain high affinity for the endoplasmic reticulum. The half-life is 14 days.

Adverse effects
Adverse effects are hot flashes, nausea, vomiting and menstrual irregularities. Tamoxifen has been identified as a hepatic carcinogen in animals; there is no clinical evidence in humans. The substance may slow the development of osteoporosis in postmenopausal women.

Clinical applications
Tamoxifen is the treatment of choice for postmenopausal women with metastatic oestrogen receptor-positive breast cancer or at high risk of recurrence, and premenopausal women with positive oestrogen receptor and tumour.

Antiandrogen (flutamide)

The chemical structure of flutamide is non-steroidal.

Mechanism of action
Flutamide is used in conjunction with gonadotropin-releasing hormone (GnRH). It inhibits the translocation of the androgen receptor from the cytoplasm to the nucleus in the hypothalamus and prostate. Indirectly it leads to increased testosterone and dihydrotestosterone production, but blocks the potential effect by inhibiting receptor translocation. The substance shows significant antitumour activity in advanced prostate cancer.

Pharmacokinetics
Fludamide is administered orally (250 mg) three times a day.

Adverse effects
Occasional side-effects are diarrhoea, nausea, vomiting and variable loss of sexual function and decreased libido.

Clinical applications
Flutamide is used for the therapy of prostate cancer.

2
Pharmacokinetically guided optimization and individualization of medical cancer chemotherapy

M. FELLHAUER and M. STARITZ

INTRODUCTION

Cancer chemotherapy drugs have a very narrow therapeutic index; therefore every effort should be made to minimize interpatient variability in drug exposure in order to maximize the benefit while keeping the risk of serious adverse effects at an acceptable level.

The need for dose individualization of drugs with a narrow therapeutic index is well accepted. For drugs that do not produce toxicity at dosages or plasma concentrations close to those required for therapeutic effects, there is little interest and need for dose optimization or individualization. In these circumstances patients are treated with dosages high enough to ensure that therapeutic concentrations are achieved. In contrast, anticancer chemotherapeutic agents, which frequently show toxicity at dosages close to those required for a therapeutic effect, provide considerable scope for dose optimization in individual patients.

When considering candidate drugs for pharmacokinetically guided dose adaptation in clinical practice the following criteria must be identified. First, a relationship must be established between plasma drug concentration and response. That means the response must be optimal in the majority of patients when plasma drug concentrations are maintained within a therapeutic range. Secondly, large interpatient variability in distribution and/or elimination of the drug is observed as a result of genetic and/or pathophysiological conditions. There may also be large differences in the sensitivity of patients to a given plasma drug concentration. Finally, another criterion may be added concerning the technical feasibility of dose adaptation.

The obvious goal of dose optimization for individual patients is to maximize the probability of producing a desired therapeutic effect while minimizing the probability of a toxic event. With anticancer drugs this goal may be modified to seek the maximum probability of producing a desired therapeutic effect while limiting toxicity.

RATIONALE FOR PHARMACOKINETICALLY GUIDED DOSE ADAPTATION

Due to the fact that pharmacokinetics of any one drug are known to be quite variable from one patient to another, both toxic and therapeutic responses to drug administration are frequently better correlated with plasma drug concentrations or the exposure of the patient to the drug (e.g. area under the plasma drug concentration–time curve (AUC)) than with the administered dose[1]. On the basis of these criteria anticancer drugs are clear candidates for pharmacokinetically guided dosage regimens, but specific problems arise. By contrast with other drugs, pharmacodynamic effects are delayed in clinical oncology: the main toxicities (neutropenia, mucositis) are observed 1 or 2 weeks after completion of treatment, and tumour response or cumulative toxicities may not be seen before multiple courses of therapy are completed.

The other important point for anticancer drugs concerns the relevance of pharmacokinetic/pharmacodynamic relationships. The relevance of the relationships between pharmacokinetics and toxicity and between pharmacokinetics and activity should be viewed in the context of the use of the drugs: for palliative treatment manageable and predictable toxicity is a primary requirement; therefore, pharmacokinetic and pharmacodynamic relationships are valuable if they can be exploited in order to achieve this. In contrast, if curative therapy is being attempted, more severe toxicity may be accepted, provided that the drug is being used to optimal therapeutic effect.

For anticancer drugs the relevant pharmacokinetic parameters for use in pharmacokinetic/pharmacodynamic relationships are generally AUC or plasma drug concentration at steady state. Other parameters are peak plasma drug concentration (C_{max}), duration of concentration above a threshold or AUC intensity.

Pharmacodynamics is here described by either discontinuous parameters (response, no response) or continuous parameters such as time to progression or survival. For toxicity, two types of parameters may also be considered: quantitative parameters such as percentage reduction in leucocyte, granulocyte or platelet counts, or semiquantitative parameters defined by World Health Organization (WHO) grading[2].

PHARMACOKINETIC–PHARMACODYNAMIC RELATIONSHIPS IN CLINICAL ONCOLOGY

Relationships between the pharmacokinetics and pharmacodynamics of anticancer drugs have been extensively reviewed. Encouraging examples of relationships between AUC and response have mainly been reported in paediatric oncology, and different strategies of pharmacokinetically guided protocols have been proposed. Moreover, examples of relationships between clinical outcome and pharmacokinetics have also been described in adults treated for solid tumours.

Many examples have been reported of the pharmacokinetic/toxicity relationships for established agents used in cancer chemotherapy. They principally concern relationships between haematological toxicity and pharmacokinetic parameters, but relationships between discontinuous parameters and pharmacokinetics have also been reported (Table 1).

Table 1 Selected clinical trials with pharmacokinetic monitoring and impact on outcome

Drug	*Disease*	*No. of patients (no. of cycles)*	*Substance measured (biological fluid)*	*Effect on outcome*
Methotrexate	ALL	108 (1503)	MTX (plasma)	CPss < 16 μmol/L ↑ relapse rate
	ALL	134 (481)	MTX (plasma)	Detection of risk factors, ↓ frequency of toxicity
	ALL	150	MTX (plasma) MTXPG (blasts)	High-dose MTX produces ↑ systemic concentrations of MTX (CPss, AUC) and ↑ concentrations of MTXPG in blasts; AUC is predictive of stomatitis; higher MTXPG is predictive of antileukaemic effects
	Osteosarcoma	97	MTX (plasma)	$Cp_{max} \geq 1000$ μmol/L predicts histological response
	Osteosarcoma	198 (1703)	MTX (plasma)	$Cp_{max} \geq 1000$ μmol/L is predictive of survival
Merceptopurine	ALL	120	6TGN (RBC)	↑ 6TGN concentrations ↑ neutropenia and survival
	ALL	172	6TGN (RBC)	↑ 6TGN concentrations ↑ disease-free survival
Methotrexate + mercaptopurine	ALL	31	6TGN and MTXPG (RBC)	↑ concentration 6TGN + MTXPG ↑ myelosuppression
	ALL	105	6TGN and MTXPG (RBC)	↑ concentration of 6TGN + MTXPG ↓ risk of relapse
Carboplatin	Ovarian cancer and sarcoma	31 (40)	Free platinum (plasma)	AUC predicted ($r = 0.89$) *a priori* based on estimation of GFR is predictive of thrombocytopenia
	Ovarian cancer	1208	None[a]	AUC was predictive of bone marrow toxicity and response rate
	Resistant or refractory cancer	24 (44)	None[a]	Thrombocytopenia predicted by dose adjusted based on BSA, renal function, and platelet counts
	Testicular carcinoma	78 (300)	None[a]	Dose adjusted based on AUC reduces risk of relapse ($p < 0.00001$)

(Continued)

Table 1 (Continued)

Drug	*Disease*	*No. of patients (no. of cycles)*	*Substance measured (biological fluid)*	*Effect on outcome*
Fluorouracil	Head and neck cancer	81 (249)	5-FU (plasma)	Dose adjustment based an mid-cycle AUC ↑ response rate while ↓ toxicity
	Head and neck cancer	186 (558)	5-FU (plasma)	Dose adjustment based an AUC ↑ response rate and survival
Teniposide	Resistant or refractory leukaemia (phase I)	28	VM-26 (plasma)	Antileukaemic response and toxicity correlated with AUC but not with dose
Etoposide	Resistant or refractory cancer	45 (90)	VP16 (plasma)	Dose adjustment based on VP-18 plasma levels ↑ treatment intensity without increasing serious toxicity
Busulfan	BMT	62	Busulfan (plasma)	Dose reduction based on mid-cycle AUC reduced the incidence of veno-occlusive disease
Suramin	Prostate cancer	37	Suramin (plasma)	Prospective dose adjustment to maintain plasma concentrations (mg/ml) within three ranges; group 1 (200–300), group 2 (175–275), group 3 (150–250); toxicity was highest in group 1, but response rate and survival similar among the three groups

Note:
[a] No substances measured in biological fluids but clearance and/or AUC estimated based on renal function. Abbreviations and symbols: ALL = acute lymphoblastic leukaemia; AUC = area under the curve; BMT = bone marrow transplant; BSA = body surface area; Cp_{max} = maximal plasma concentration; CPss = plasma concentration at steady state, 5-FU = fluorouracil, GFR = glomerular filtration rate; 6-MP = mercaptopurine; MTX = methotrexate; MTXPG = methotrexate polyglutamate (intracellular MTX active metabolites); RBC = red blood cells; 6TGN = 8 thioguanine nucleotides (intracellular 6-MP active metabolites); VM-26 = teniposide; VP-16 = etoposide; ↑ = increase; ↓ = decrease.

METHODS OF DRUG DOSAGE ADJUSTMENT IN CLINICAL ONCOLOGY

Conventional method

Traditionally, anticancer drugs have been standardized to body surface area (BSA) or body weight; this practice is based on the relationship that exists between body size (e.g. total body weight and BSA) and physiological functions such as cardiac output, liver or renal blood flow and glomerular filtration rate. The BSA is particularly useful for scaling between infants and adults and to adapt the dose for obese patients. The goal of dose standardization is to provide consistent systemic drug exposure. The nomogram most commonly used in clinical practice to estimate BSA was derived in 1916 by DuBois and DuBois from only nine non-obese individuals of varying age, shape and size. This formula remains the most appropriate method of estimating BSA. It was challenged in 1970 by Gehen and George who directly measured the skin-surface

Table 2 Practical methods of drug adjustment in clinical oncology

Drug	*Method of dose adjustment*	*Criteria*	*Objectives*
Anthracyclines	*A priori*	Liver function (bilirubin)	Risk of major toxicity
Carboplatin	*A priori*	Renal function: GFR	Target AUC with maximum likelihood of toxicity
Docetaxel	*A priori*	BSA	Efficacy and minimum likelihood of toxicity
Etoposide	*A priori* *A priori* During continuous infusion	Liver function (enzymes) Renal function Css	Risk of major neutropenia Limit major toxicity Obtain maximum likelihood of efficacy and minimum likelihood of toxicity
Fluorouracil	*A priori* During continuous infusion	DPD deficiency	Avoid life-threatening toxicity AUC at mid-cycle; obtain maximum and minimum likelihood of toxicity
	During repeated administration	Css	Obtain maximum likelihood of efficacy and minimum likelihood of toxicity
Mercaptopurine	*A priori* During repeated administration	TPMT deficiency Erythrocyte thioguanine nucleotides	Avoid life-threatening toxicity Control treatment compliance
Methotrexate	Adaptive rescue	C_{min} 24 h and 48 h after infusion	Avoid life-threatening toxicity or minimize likelihood of toxicity

AUC = area under the plasma drug concentration–time curve; BSA = body surface area; C_{min} = trough plasma drug concentration; Css = Plasma drug concentration at steady state; DPD = dihydropyrimidine dehydrogenase; TPMT = thiopurine methyltransferase.

area of 401 individuals and surprisingly confirmed the validity of the nomogram. The usefulness of adopting anticancer drug dose to BSA in adults has been questioned. A retrospective analysis of more than 300 patients and nine anticancer agents caused doubt as to whether normalization of doses to BSA is of sufficient clinical value in achieving consistent drug exposure.

Additionally the number of drugs for which clearance has been poorly correlated with BSA, or not correlated at all, has grown. Despite this clear demonstration, the practice of dosage adjustment to BSA is so widespread that it may be difficult to change it to a more rational approach. It is necessary to consider that heavy and tall people presenting with a large BSA do not necessarily have a better function of liver or kidneys.

In practice most agents were used in a mg/m^2 or mg/kg dose recommended for phase II trials. This recommended dose is based on the results of phase I clinical trials and its recommendation usually involves no pharmacokinetic consideration. Dose reductions or delays are implemented in patients developing unacceptable toxicity, but doses are seldom escalated in the absence of toxicity. As a result of the poor therapeutic indexes of anticancer drugs, this means that patients not showing signs of toxicity are receiving lower doses than possible.

A-priori dosage determination based on patient characteristics

Dose adaptation attempts to take into account patient characteristics known to affect the pharmacokinetics or pharmacodynamics of an anticancer drug. As with other agents, hepatic and renal function must be explored before administration of anticancer drugs. While renal dysfunction is easily evaluated by measuring serum creatinine level or calculating creatinine clearance (CL_{CR}) the impact of hepatic dysfunction on drug elimination or metabolism is more difficult to determine. The major problem is that hepatic enzymes and serum bilirubin levels are insufficient indicators of metabolizing activity. Moreover, alternating hepatic function tests, such as indocyanine green (a marker of hepatic blood flow), phenazone (a substrate marker for cytochrome P450 activity) or lorazepam (a substrate marker of hepatic glucuronidation) show limited value in predicting the pharmacokinetics of chemotherapeutic drugs, and are not yet clinically established. More different guidelines for the characteristics of anticancer drugs are unfortunately not available. Thus the value of *a-priori* dosage determination based on patient characteristics remains limited.

Dose adaptation according to renal or liver function

Carboplatin

Carboplatin is mainly eliminated by the kidneys. About 65% of the administered dose is recovered in the urine, mostly as unchanged carboplatin 24 h after administration. Calvert et al.[3] showed that renal clearance of carboplatin is related directly to the GFR, but poorly to the BSA. The non-renal clearance consisting of protein and tissue binding represents one-quarter of total body clearance when renal function is normal. The total body clearance of carboplatin is highly variable from one individual to another and ranges between 20 and 200 ml/min. Moreover, the carboplatin AUC to which a patient is exposed correlates with carboplatin-induced thrombocytopenia. This occurs when the drug is given as a single agent and when it is given in combination with cyclophosphamide, etoposide or paclitaxel. Differences were observed between patients previously treated with chemotherapy and those who were untreated. A correlation between duration of leucocyte nadir and carboplatin AUC is also known in high-dose regimens and in combination therapy with either etoposide, fluorouracil or paclitaxel, or with both vinblastine and methotrexate. In different studies no relationship could be demonstrated between carboplatin dose and degree of thrombocytopenia, although a good correlation with carboplatin AUC was obvious[4]. All these data suggest that the AUC in the individual patient is the most important factor in predicting the degree of thrombocytopenia and leucopenia with carboplatin. AUC is an important determinant of the therapeutic effect of carboplatin.

The retrospective calculation of AUC has also been used to study its effect on myelosuppression and response rate in ovarian cancer. Jodrell et al.[5] studied 1028 patients with ovarian cancer treated in phase II studies with carboplatin. In these patients the GFR was either retrospectively estimated by the Cockcroft–Gault equation or prospectively determined by [^{51}Cr]ethylene diamine tetra-acetic acid (^{51}Cr EDTA) clearance. AUC was then estimated from the total dose of carboplatin given. This study demonstrated that, for both untreated and previously treated patients, the response rate increased as the AUC increased up to 5 mg/ml per minute. A further increase in the AUC beyond this point resulted in little further increase in the response rate, suggesting that there was a plateau in the AUC-response effect. However, further studies did not confirm the existence of this plateau: in a prospective randomized trial in ovarian cancer the administration of chemotherapy to achieve an AUC of 12 mg/ml per minute every 4 weeks (for four cycles) was associated with a complete response rate of 58%, whereas an AUC of 6 mg/ml per minute every 4 weeks for six courses produced a response rate of only 32%. Different approaches to the determination of carboplatin dosage include the following:

Thrombocyte nadir-directed dosage During phase I clinical trials Egorin et al.[6] developed an approach to individualizing carboplatin dosage. They demonstrated first that the clearance of carboplatin was related to the GFR determined by CL_{CR}, and secondly that the degree of thrombocytopenia was related to the carboplatin AUC. They derived from these observations a formula by which the dose of carboplatin could be calculated on the basis of the measured pretreatment CL_{CR}, the patient's BSA and the desired thrombocyte nadir. A separate formula was calculated for patients previously exposed to myelosuppressive therapy.

In non-pretreated patients:

$$\text{Dosage (mg/m}^2) = (0.091)\frac{CL_{CR}}{BSA}\left(\frac{PPC - PND}{PPC} \times 100\right) + 86 \qquad (1)$$

where BSA = body surface area, CL_{CR} = measured creatinine clearance, PND = platelet nadir desired and PPC = pretreatment platelet count.

In pretreated patients:

$$\text{Dosage (mg/m}^2\text{)} = (0.091)\frac{\text{CL}_{\text{CR}}}{\text{BSA}}\left(\left[\frac{\text{PPC} - \text{PND}}{\text{PPC}} \times 100\right] - 17\right) + 86 \qquad (2)$$

This formula was prospectively validated in a study which confirmed that the observed thrombocyte nadirs correlated closely with the desired values[7].

This formula allows the clinician to calculate the dose on the basis of the clinical endpoint thrombocytopenia. However, in some combination regimens thrombocytopenia may not be the pharmacodynamic endpoint that is of interest, since neutropenia may have caused the dose-limiting toxicity.

AUC-directed dosage Calvert et al.[3] have developed a formula to allow a dose of carboplatin to be calculated in order to achieve a targeted AUC:

$$\text{Dose (mg carboplatin)} = \text{AUC (mg/ml per minute)} \times (\text{GFR} + 25)\ \text{(ml/min)} \qquad (3)$$

The formula has been validated in a prospective study[3]. In these studies the GFR was determined by isotopic measurement of [^{51}Cr]EDTA clearance.

The feasibility of obtaining rapid and reliable estimates of GFR is indeed a problem, particularly when isotopic determination is not available. In clinical practice, estimation of GFR is possible using plasma creatinine levels according to the Cockcroft–Gault or Jeliffe equations. Both formulas correlate with the [^{51}Cr]EDTA method, but they are biased: both underpredict the GFR for high carboplatin clearances and overpredict it for low CL_{CR}. These biases result in patients being exposed to a lower AUC than expected when their GFR exceeds 50–60 ml/min, or to a higher AUC when their GFR is lower. The degree of underprediction increases as the GFR increases.

Another possibility for estimating GFR consists of 24-h urinary creatinine. This biochemical determination shows discrepancies if accurate figures of the 24-h urinary collection are not confirmed. Finally, the approach of using population pharmacokinetics of carboplatin has been attempted, investigating the relationship between carboplatin clearance and a number of factors including the plasma creatinine level. Age, weight, sex and serum creatinine level were significant independent variables in determining carboplatin clearance and the 'Chatelut formula' allows carboplatin clearance to be calculated directly[8]:

$$\text{CL}_{\text{carbo}}\ \text{(ml/min)} = 0.134\,\text{BW} + \frac{218 \times \text{BW} \times (1 - 0.00457 \times \text{age}) \times [1 - (0.314 \times \text{gender})]}{\text{serum creatinine } (\mu\text{mol/L})} \qquad (4)$$

where CL_{carbo} = carboplatin clearance, BW = bodyweight, and gender = 0 if male and 1 if female. This formula showed a little bias and a precision similar to that of the [^{51}Cr]EDTA method. It seems that *a-priori* estimation of carboplatin clearance is highly dependent on the biochemical method for determination of serum creatinine level.

Target AUC of carboplatin in monotherapy and in combined regimens Target AUC is defined as a function of the combination of drugs used. When carboplatin is used as a single agent, an AUC of 7 mg/ml per minute should be targeted when the patient is chemotherapy-naive. In combination with etoposide, cyclophosphamide or vinorelbine, this AUC should be reduced to 5 mg/ml per minute. Because of a pharmacodynamic interaction between paclitaxel and carboplatin (decrease of carboplatin-induced thrombocytopenia), an AUC of 7 mg/ml per minute for carboplatin could be reached. In pretreated patients an AUC of 5–4 mg/ml per minute is recommended in monochemotherapy as well as in combination. The use of these different approaches for dose determination is valid for AUC lower than 2 mg/ml per minute which are usually targeted when carboplatin is combined with radiotherapy.

Etoposide

Etoposide is a semi-synthetic epipodophyllotoxin. The toxicity of this drug has been shown to be regimen-dependent. Its pharmacokinetics have been intensively studied in a wide variety of patient groups with different regimens, alone or in combination with other chemotherapeutic agents.

The pharmacokinetics of etoposide are linear over a large range of doses. The drug is extensively bound to plasma protein. It is eliminated by both renal and biliary pathways mainly as unchanged etoposide. Relationships have been established between total or free etoposide AUC and neutropenia, which represents the dose-limiting toxicity in monochemotherapy and in combination.

Impaired renal function

Patients with impaired renal function objectivated by serum creatinine levels greater than the normal range experienced significantly worse haematological toxicity than patients with normal renal function. A dose reduction of approximately one-third is sufficient to correct this increase in AUC and result in a drug exposure similar to that in patients with normal renal function. The cut-off serum creatinine amounts to 130 μmol/L. Moreover, a population pharmacokinetic study performed in 100 patients proposed a formula to determine the decrease in renal clearance as a function of serum creatinine levels. This population approach proposed a relationship between serum creatinine levels and etoposide clearance. Consequently, a more rational adaptation of etoposide dosage was proposed in the case of renal dysfunction.

Impaired liver function

In the case of impaired liver function, different types of patients must be considered. The role of the liver in etoposide clearance may actually be as important as renal clearance. Approximately 50% of an intravenous dose of ^{14}C-labelled etoposide was recovered in the faeces of cancer patients. Moreover, it is important to take into account the impact of liver dysfunction on serum albumin levels. In patients with hyperbilirubinaemia serum bilirubin influences protein binding of the drug. Thus in patients with hyperbilirubinaemia the dose should be reduced by 30%.

Taxanes
Paclitaxel is a diterpenoid taxane derivative. The dose-limiting toxicity of the drug is neutropenia. Paclitaxel displays nonlinear pharmacokinetics, particularly at shorter infusion times and at high doses. Hepatic metabolism and biliary excretion are the most important elimination routes of paclitaxel and its metabolites. The total faecal excretion is approximately 70% of the administered dose, with 6α-hydroxy-paclitaxel being the major component in most patients. Thus, it can be expected that the pharmacokinetics and pharmacodynamics of paclitaxel differ in patients with impaired liver function. Some small studies have demonstrated that paclitaxel can be safely given at normal doses to patients with mild liver dysfunction (normal bilirubin and transaminases less than 10 times normal values). In patients with elevated bilirubin levels no guidelines are available in the literature.

Docetaxel is another new semisynthetic taxoid. The dose-limiting toxicities of docetaxel consist of neutropenia and peripheral neurotoxicity. Docetaxel exhibits linear pharmacokinetics characterized by a three-compartment model; it is mainly eliminated by metabolism and biliary excretion. The proportion of the dose excreted in urine is only 10%; therefore the pharmacokinetics of this drug are not affected by impaired renal function. A good correlation was found between docetaxel AUC and neutropenia. Population pharmacokinetic/pharmacodynamic studies of single-agent docetaxel were prospectively performed; they demonstrated that docetaxel clearance was highly correlated with BSA, justifying a dosage for that drug calculated in mg/m^2. Moreover, the population studies have identified five covariables (age > 70 years, hypoalbuminaemia, elevation of α_1-acid glycoprotein, low α_1-acid glycoprotein levels and elevated levels of the liver enzymes ALT and AST which are predictive for a reduced clearance. As a correlation was found between docetaxel clearance and the risk of severe neutropenia, these parameters allow identification of patients at high risk of severe neutropenia. Consequently a rational dosage reduction is possible.

Anthracyclines
The anthracycline antibiotics, daunorubicin, doxorubicin, epirubicin and idarubicin, are rapidly and extensively metabolized following systemic administration. The primary metabolites include daunorubicinol, doxorubicinol, epirubicinol, idarubicinol and various glucuroconjugated or aglycone metabolites. The urinary excretion of these compounds and their metabolites, measured for 4 or 5 days following drug administration, accounted for less than 20% of the dose. Thus, there is no pharmacokinetic basis for the dosage adjustment of the anthracycline antibiotics in the presence of impaired renal function.

In the case of impaired hepatic function it is proposed for doxorubicin to reduce the dosage as a function of serum bilirubin level and serum liver enzyme level. When bilirubin levels exceeded 12–50 mg/L it was recommended to reduce the doxorubicin dose by 50–75%, or to stop altogether.

Topotecan
Topotecan, an analogue of camptothecin, is an inhibitor of DNA topoisomerase I. The urinary recovery of topotecan ranges from 40% to 70%, suggesting that renal excretion is the primary clearance pathway. A recent study including

patients with normal and impaired renal function showed significant correlation between systemic plasma clearance of topotecan and CL_{CR}. In patients with mild renal dysfunction (CL_{CR} ranging from 40 to 60 ml/min), no dose adjustment is required. By contrast, in patients with moderate renal impairment (CL_{CR} of < 40 ml/min), a dose reduction by 50% is recommended. In patients with impaired hepatic function the nature and severity of toxic effects and the pharmacokinetics of topotecan were similar to those observed in patients with normal hepatic function. Cancer patients with hepatic injury can be treated with topotecan without dose modification.

Vinca alkaloids

Vinca alkaloid derivatives (vincristine, vinblastine, vindesine, vinorelbine) are not excreted significantly in the urine. Dosage adjustment is not necessary for vinca alkaloids in patients with renal impairment. Various studies have investigated the impact of liver disorders on the pharmacokinetics of vincristine. Reduced clearance was associated with raised serum alkaline phosphatase. However, guidelines for dosage adjustment are not yet available.

Vinorelbine is a vinca alkaloid; its pharmacokinetics have been studied in breast cancer patients with liver metastases. Vinorelbine clearance was significantly reduced in patients with massive metastatic liver involvement in whom more than 75% of liver volume was replaced by tumour and high levels of bilirubin, transaminases and γ-glutamyl transferase. Moreover, its clearance is significantly correlated with the monoethylglycinexylidide test ($r^2 = 0.7$; $p < 0.0001$) which might be useful for individualization of the vinorelbine dosage. Patients with large metastatic liver involvement should receive reduced doses not exceeding 30% of normal doses.

Melphalan

Melphalan is an alkylating agent. The drug is both secreted and reabsorbed by the renal tubules. The mean urinary excretion of unchanged melphalan ranges from 15% to 98%. Some studies have recommended a dose reduction in patients with renal impairment, and a positive correlation of melphalan clearance with GFR has been reported. A careful follow-up of haematological toxicity and possibly a dose reduction of melphalan are proposed for myeloma patients with renal impairment.

Dose adaptation in the elderly

The question of whether age is a reason for modification of pharmacokinetic parameters has received no clear and definitive answer; in fact ageing cannot be considered as an independent feature, and is characterized by a conjunction of physiological changes that may occur together. These changes include hypoalbuminaemia due to poor nutrition, reduction of hepatic or renal blood flow, decreased body mass index, impaired hepatic and renal function and several other conditions. Recently, age was identified as the patient feature which had the greatest impact on fluorouracil clearance compared with other covariables. Only very few specific studies have been performed concerning the pharmacokinetics of anticancer drugs in elderly patients. It therefore appears that dose adaptation as a function of individual physiology is better than adaptation as a function of chronological age.

Dose adaptation in the obese patient

As mentioned above, doses of anticancer drugs have been standardized to BSA. Selecting drug doses can be a challenging decision for the clinician when treating a cancer patient who is significantly overweight. If total body weight is used to determine BSA, calculated doses can be as much as 25–30% higher than if ideal body weight is used, with the potential for severe toxicity. Up to now no dosage guidelines have been established for obese patients receiving cancer chemotherapy. However, a limitation of calculated BSA at a level of 2.2 m^2 is usually recommended. Obese persons show changes of normal physiology, increase in blood volume, cardiac output, lean body mass, organ size and adipose tissue mass. Only very few studies have reported the influence of body fatness on the pharmacokinetics of antineoplastic drugs. These studies collectively suggest that differences exist in the pharmacokinetics of anticancer agents between patients with normal body weight and obese patients, but these differences may be difficult to objectivate and characterize adequately. Finally, obesity must be taken into account when predicting the clearance of drugs such as carboplatin. Benezet et al.[9] demonstrated that actual body weight must be balanced by ideal body weight to estimate clearance using the Chatelut formula.

Pharmacogenetics

Recent developments in the field of pharmacogenetics should also be noted in the context of dose adaptation. Some drugs require metabolism to be activated or inactivated. Some enzymes involved in the biotransformation have polymorphic expression; therefore, assessing enzyme activity (i.e. phenotype) or gene mutations (i.e. genotype) could help to predict optimal dose regimens.

Fluorouracil is catabolized into dihydrofluorouracil (5-FUH2) by dihydropyrimidine dehydrogenase (DPD). Patients who are genetically deficient in this enzyme are at particular risk of life-threatening toxicity. The gene for DPD has recently been localized to chromosome lp22, and at least one mutation has been identified. For all other patients who are not genetically deficient there seems to be no case for adjusting doses on the basis of the variations in the normal levels of this enzyme.

Mercaptopurine is sometimes applied in conjunction with methotrexate. The influence of pharmacogenetics and variability in metabolism of the pharmacology of mercaptopurine is now well documented. This drug is inactivated by *S*-methylation, a reaction catalysed by the enzyme thiopurine methyltransferase (TPMT). A polymorphic variation in the activity of this enzyme has been described. Deficiency in TPMT, due to homozygosity for low TPMT, is quite rare (1 in 300), but can lead to pronounced toxicity. TPMT activity varies widely in the subpopulation who have intermediate TPMT activity and can be related inversely to formation of the active 6-thioguanine nucleotide (6-TGN) metabolites and therapeutic response. Finally, homozygotes for high TPMT activity may be resistant to mercaptopurine therapy and can tolerate high doses of the drug, without experiencing myelosuppression. Individualization of mercaptopurine dose, based on TPMT activity, is a good example of the use of a patient characteristic to optimize drug administration.

Many anticancer drugs are extensively metabolized by CYP enzymes, especially the isoenzymes CYP3A4 and CYP2C8. Cyclophosphamide, ifosfamide, taxol, docetaxel, irinotecan, epipodophyllotoxins and vinca alkaloids are especially metabolized by these enzymes. Even though there is no evidence of polymorphism in these enzymes, a large variability of their activity has been observed in humans. Moreover, significant clinical interactions have been described due to inhibitors or activators of these enzymes in clinical oncology. For example, the concomitant use of anticonvulsant drugs with paclitaxel led to an increase in the maximum tolerated use of paclitaxel because of a modification in the metabolism profile.

The UDP glycosyltransferases (UGTs) represent a superfamily of enzymes that catalyse addition of the glycosyl group from a nucleotide sugar to a hydrophobic molecule. This is the case for irinotecan, which is activated by a carboxylesterase to form the active metabolite SN-38, a potent inhibitor of topoisomerase. SN-38 is further conjugated by UGT. Recently it was shown that the UGT 1A1 isoform is responsible for the glucuronidation of SN-38. The same isoform conjugates bilirubin or several endogenous substrates. Moreover, when hepatic microsomes from patients who have Criggler–Najjar type I syndrome were incubated with SN-38, a very important deficit in glucuronidation was observed, suggesting a genetic predisposition to the metabolism of irinotecan and an increased risk of irinotecan toxicity. It should be mentioned that a recent study showed that patients with Gilbert syndrome treated with irinotecan experienced severe toxicity. These authors suggest that unconjugated serum bilirubin could be a predictive parameter for irinotecan toxicity.

Dose adaptation during repeated or continuous administration

Duration of drug infusion offers a simple method of dose adaptation. For drugs with one-compartment pharmacokinetics, 90% of the full concentration is reached within three half-lives of the substance. When a stable plasma concentration is reached and determined, it is possible to modify the infusion rate for the remainder of the course of treatment if a relationship has been established between plasma level and a pharmacodynamic endpoint. This methodology has been used for continuous intravenous infusions of fluorouracil and etoposide. However, it is also applicable to repeated oral administration of drugs such as etoposide or to repeated weekly intravenous administration of fluorouracil or cisplatin.

Another possibility for dose adaptation consists of administering a low test dose of an anticancer drug to determine exactly the pharmacokinetic parameter for the individual patient, and then modifying the dose to obtain a target AUC. Such a method has been used for methotrexate and melphalan. Though these attempts are possible they are not really clinically established.

Fluorouracil

Fluorouracil is one of the oldest drugs used in cancer chemotherapy. Despite its extensive use in the treatment of gastrointestinal tumours, its pharmacokinetics remain complex because of the existence of both dose- and time-dependence. A relationship was demonstrated between toxicity and the explosure of patients to the drug when it was administered by continuous infusion for 3–5 days in association with cisplatin. There is evidence that the AUC obtained at midcycle predicts the development of fluorouracil-induced stomatitis. Consequently, nomograms have been developed to adjust the dose of fluorouracil based on its plasma concentrations. Adaptation of the dose at mid-cycle resulted in a decrease in the incidence of stomatitis from 20% to 12%. In addition, a better response was observed in patients with dosage adjustments even though no upward adjustment was made. Response rate and patient survival may correlate with fluorouracil AUC but not with the dose.

Another method is to use a dosage-adjustment strategy: investigations showed that a weekly 8-h intravenous infusion of high-dose fluorouracil (1.3 g/m^2) with folinic acid produced the best response rates with acceptable toxicity when plasma concentrations were between 2 and 3 mg/L. The acute toxicity of different types was correlated with plasma fluorouracil concentrations higher than 3 mg/L and not with the overall dose. This dosage adjustment led to an increase in dose intensity of fluorouracil in metastatic colorectal cancer.

In a recent prospective trial there was evidence that individual dose adjustment with pharmacokinetic monitoring (dose ranging from 950 to 3400 mg/m^2 per week) provided high survival and response rates with good tolerability.

Etoposide

The phase-specific nature of etoposide cytotoxicity is well documented. Pharmacokinetic studies performed during these clinical trials also suggested that plasma etoposide concentrations associated with haematological toxicities (2–3 mg/L) were higher than those associated with antitumour activity (1–2 mg/L). Despite the limited stability of etoposide in aqueous solution, several groups have investigated the use of continuous infusion of etoposide. Those studies showed that the dose-limiting toxicity of etoposide (neutropenia) is highly correlated with the degree of systemic exposure of unbound drug.

Recently investigators have developed another strategy based an a target Css of etoposide after a loading dose administered prior to a 5-day continuous infusion. Haematological toxicity was higher in patients with a Css reaching 3 mg/L than in patients with a figure of 2 mg/L. Equally important was the demonstration that tumour response was similar in the two cohorts of patients with small-cell lung cancer. Moreover, the target Css was reached with a very low confidence limit. Such differences between toxicity and tumour response as a function of plasma concentrations have been recently reported when a 14-day infusion of etoposide was used. Therapeutic monitoring of infused etoposide is feasible and helps to overcome problems associated with pharmacokinetic variability. The difference between the doses required for obtaining maximum antitumour response and toxicity suggest that these two pharmacodynamic effects may be associated with the maintenance of target plasma concentrations.

Another alternative for continuous exposure to etoposide was the use of the oral formulation; however, the inter- and intra-patient variability in bioavailability with oral etoposide is likely to contribute to the unpredictable toxicity seen in some patients. This makes the estimation of total systemic exposure over a course of treatment, or dose optimization in individual patients based on AUC or a specific plasma concentration, difficult to achieve.

Methotrexate

Methotrexate is an antifolate. Plasma drug concentrations have been shown to be the best predictor for methotrexate toxicity. Consequently, the monitoring of methotrexate concentrations in plasma is now routinely performed to predict which patients will require folinic acid rescue and to adapt the dose of this antidote. The use of very high doses of methotrexate in children has stimulated the development of a test dose for determining the dosage necessary to reach a plasma concentration of 10^{-5} mol/L for a 36-h infusion or of 10^{-3} mol/L for an 8-h infusion.

More recently, cellular levels of methotrexate and its polyglutamated derivatives have been measured and related to clinical effect. Polyglutamated intracellular metabolites of methotrexate are more active inhibitors of the target enzyme dihydrofolate reductase than the parenteral compound. Large inter- and intra-patient variation in the concentrations of these polyglutamates has been reported. The clinical consequence of this finding has not yet been investigated.

Dose adaptation with feedback control

The approach of adaptive dosage with feedback control is the most complicated and complex method. Though these attempts are established in principle, they are not yet clinically established.

CONCLUSIONS

A better knowledge of drug pharmacokinetics and pharmacodynamics contributes to optimization and individualization of anticancer drug therapy. The routine use of pharmacokinetic methods in determining the dosage of carboplatin, methotrexate, fluorouracil or etoposide indicates that such optimization is feasible. For these drugs the concept of AUC-based dosage has been validated since toxicities are clearly related to the AUC. Moreover, it seems likely that therapeutic efficacy is also related to AUC, although further clinical trials are necessary to establish this point clearly. Whereas therapeutic drug monitoring in all patients is not yet established clinically, the routine use of BSA for calculating the dosage should be avoided. Methods which are based on the pharmacological characteristics of the drug and the personal characteristics of the patient are to be preferred.

For anticancer agents with a very narrow therapeutic index every effort should be made to minimize inter-patient variability in drug exposure in order to maximize the benefit while keeping the risk of serious adverse effects at an acceptable level.

References

1. Moore MJ, Erlichman C. Therapeutic drug monitoring in oncology: problems and potential in antineoplastic therapy. Clin Pharmacokinet. 1987;13:205–7.
2. Egorin MJ, Reyno LM, Canetta RM et al. Modeling toxicity and response in carboplatin-based combination chemotherapy. Semin Oncol. 1994;5(Suppl.12):7–19.
3. Calvert AH, Newell DR, Gumbrell LA et al. Carboplatin dosage; prospective evaluation of a simple formula based on renal function. J Clin Oncol. 1989;7:1748–56.
4. Chatelut E, Chevreau C, Brunner V et al. A pharmacologically guided phase I study of carboplatin in combination with methotrexate and vinblastine in advanced urothelial cancer. Cancer Chemother Pharmacol. 1995;35:391–6.
5. Jodrell D, Egorin MJ, Canetta RM. Relationships between carboplatin exposure and tumor response and toxicity in patients with ovarian cancer. J Clin Oncol. 1992;10:520–8.
6. Egorin MJ, Van Echo DA, Tipping SJ et al. Pharmacokinetics and dosage reduction of cis-diammine (1,1-cyclobutanedicarboxylato)platinum in patients with impaired renal function. Cancer Res. 1984;44:5432–8.
7. Egorin MJ, Van Echo DA, Olman EA et al. Prospective validation of a pharmacologically based dosing scheme for the cis-diamminedichloroplatinum (II) analogue diamminecyclobutanedicarboxylatoplatinum. Cancer Res. 1985;45:6502–6.
8. Chatelut E, Canal P, Brunner V et al. Prediction of carboplatin clearance from standard morphological and biological patient characteristics. J Natl Cancer Inst. 1995;87:573–80.
9. Benezet S, Guimbaud R, Chatelut E et al. How to predict carboplatin clearance from standard morphological and biological characteristics in obese patients. Ann Oncol. 1997;8:607–9.

3
Pharmacokinetics of anticancer agents in patients with impaired liver function*

M.G. DONELLI, M. ZUCCHETTI, E. MUNZONE, M. D'INCALCI and A. CROSIGNANI

INTRODUCTION

Liver disease may have a substantial and unpredictable effect on drug kinetics by: (1) altering the intrinsic hepatic clearance; (2) reducing the metabolic capacity of the liver; (3) affecting excretion into the bile; (4) reducing the production of albumin thus decreasing serum, protein binding and increasing the fraction of free compound; and (5) affecting absorption from the gastrointestinal tract in cases of severe portal hypertension. Reduced hepatic clearance may be due to reduced hepatocellular uptake and, if concomitant portal hypertension and portosystemic shunts are present, to reduced liver blood flow.

In cancer patients liver dysfunction may result from other diseases affecting the liver such as hepatitis or cirrhosis, from toxicity induced by chemotherapy or from deterioration of liver function in the presence of a neoplastic process which reduces the functioning, metabolizing liver mass. Impaired drug clearance may be due to a decreased liver cell mass, to a reduced metabolizing capacity of the hepatocyte or finally to a reduction of hepatic blood flow due to metastases compressing liver tissue.

Liver dysfunction may be important because of changes in the metabolism of anticancer drugs which undergo hepatic biotransformation, either producing active metabolites (e.g. cyclophosphamide, dacarbazine) or resulting in detoxified products (e.g. doxorubicin, mitoxantrone, vinca alkaloids). For drugs which are highly protein-bound (e.g. etoposide or anthracycline antibiotics), a condition of hypoalbuminaemia, which may result from severely impaired liver

* Reprinted from: *European Journal of Cancer*, Vol. 34, pages 33–46 © 1998 Elsevier Ltd., with permission from Elsevier.

function, together with concomitant hyperbilirubinaemia, which may be due to both severe liver impairment and severe cholestasis, may increase the fraction of unbound drug responsible for therapeutic and toxic effects[1–3].

Increased toxicity, sometimes associated with delayed drug clearance, has been described for a series of anticancer agents[4,5] in patients with several biochemical indicators of liver dysfunction. To avoid toxicity, drastic dose reductions have often been suggested, but underdosage risks reducing the efficacy of the drug. There is a lack of reliable dosage modification schemes, based on detailed pharmacological studies in patients with liver disease.

Patient population studies are not homogeneous and often no detailed diagnosis is reported. In addition, information on the ultrasonographic and endoscopic signs of portal hypertension and on liver histology is only rarely reported. Therefore, the clinical data considered so far for their relationship with pharmacokinetic parameters are limited to biochemical indices, which unfortunately reflect a wide variety of pathophysiological changes.

This chapter reviews the literature on the clinical pharmacokinetics of the most widely used antitumour agents, such as anthracycline antibiotics and analogues, alkylating agents, antimetabolites, epipodophyllotoxins, vinca alkaloids and taxanes, for which the question of dosage adjustment has been raised when a tumour involves the liver, or liver function tests are altered. Since in most studies the patients had mild or moderate liver dysfunction, resulting in only slight changes of the biochemical tests, it was not possible to relate modification of the pharmacokinetic profile with the degree of liver dysfunction.

Published studies were identified through a computer search for the period 1973–1996 using the Medline database of the National Library of Medicine (Bethesda, Maryland, USA) and by inspecting the bibliographies of original and review articles on the pharmacology of antitumour agents in patients with abnormal liver function.

LIVER FUNCTION TESTS

The most commonly used liver function tests were serum biochemical indices. These tests, listed in Table 1, reflect a variety of pathophysiological changes of different degrees. For example, serum transaminases, ALT (alanine aminotransferase) or SGPT (serum glutamic pyruvic transaminase), and AST (aspartate aminotransferase) or SGOT (serum glutamic oxaloacetic transaminase) mainly reflect the degree of liver inflammation and are consequently related to hepatocellular necrosis. Therefore, it is not correct to employ AST and ALT as indices of liver function, and in any case no quantitative relationship can be established between liver function impairment and changes in serum transaminases. Serum bilirubin levels are mostly related to severe cholestasis or severe liver impairment. However, this parameter lacks sensitivity, since serum bilirubin rises only if there is very severe impairment[6]. 'The test also lacks specificity since it is also elevated in haematological conditions and in subjects with congenitally deficient hepatic conjugation'[6]. This condition, known as Gilbert's syndrome, is highly prevalent in the general population, so it is questionable whether a mild increase of total bilirubin truly reflects impairment of liver function. Cholestasis may markedly affect the pharmacokinetics of drugs which are significantly excreted in the bile, and impaired liver function is also associated with reduced hepatic uptake and metabolism.

Reduced production of albumin, increased prothrombin time or serum pseudocholinesterase levels are other parameters widely used to measure liver function roughly. However, these were used very seldom in the papers reviewed.

Dynamic liver function tests such as the antipyrine test, galactose elimination capacity, bromosulphthalein clearance and, recently, the mono-ethylglycine-xylidide test based on lidocaine metabolite formation[7,8], would be more appropriate to evaluate liver function quantitatively. However, they are not widely

Table 1 Pathophysiological significance of altered biochemical indices associated with liver dysfunction and their utility in assessing and quantifying liver impairment

Biochemical indices	*Normal serum levels*	*Underlying patho-physiological condition*	*Limitations for clinical use*	*Relationship with impairment of liver function*
Bilirubin	<1.2 mg/100 ml	Severe cholestasis Impaired liver function	Low sensitivity Low specificity	†Moderate: 2–3 mg/100 ml †Severe: >3 mg/100 ml
Transaminase:	*<45 U.I./L	Inflammation	Unrelated to liver function	No quantitative relationship
Alanine amino-transferase (ALT)		Cytolysis		
Aspartate amino-transferase (AST)				
Alkaline phos-phatase (APH)	*<279 U.I./L	Cholestasis	Unrelated to liver function	No quantitative relationship
γ-Glutamyl transferase	*<32 U.I./L in	Cholestasis	Unrelated to liver function	No quantitative relationship
(γ-GT)	*<50 U.I./L in			
Pseudocho-linesterase (CHE)	> 4600 U.I./L	Impaired liver function	Rough measure of liver function; wide range of normality	Not well established
Albumin	>3.5 g/100 ml	Impaired liver function	Rough measure of liver function; influenced by nutrition	†Moderate: 3–3.5 g/100 ml †Severe: < 3.0 g/100 ml
Prothrombin activity	80–100%	Impaired liver function	Rough measure of liver function; influenced by cholestasis	†Moderate: 40–70% †Severe: < 40%

* Most widely used range.

† Moderate and severe impairment of liver function were defined on the basis of the widely used Child-Pugh classification of liver cirrhosis [93J]. ALT, SGPT (serum glutamic pyruvic transaminase); AST, SGOT (serum glutamic oxaloacetic transaminase).

used in clinical practice, because they are laborious, and were evaluated in only a few of the studies reviewed.

DOXORUBICIN

For doxorubicin (DOX) and all the anthracyclines that are primarily metabolized and excreted by the liver (Figure 1), pharmacokinetic alterations should be expected to be related to abnormal liver function, as in experimental animals[9]. The drug that has been most widely investigated in this regard is DOX, and Table 2 summarizes the main reports describing its pharmacokinetic behaviour in cancer patients with hepatic impairment.

The conventional guideline for clinical practice is mostly based on the early reports by Benjamin and associates[10,11] describing elimination of DOX in the presence of liver disease, evaluated on the basis of serum bilirubin levels. However, these papers, which raised the question of liver function impairment in cancer therapy, suffer from many limitations, since they give few details on the pharmacology studies and make no mention of other liver function tests. The studies reported deal with eight patients with abnormal bilirubin levels. Three had serum bilirubin higher than 3 mg/100 ml, with severe pancytopenia and painful mucositis, and three drug-related deaths were observed. As plasma levels

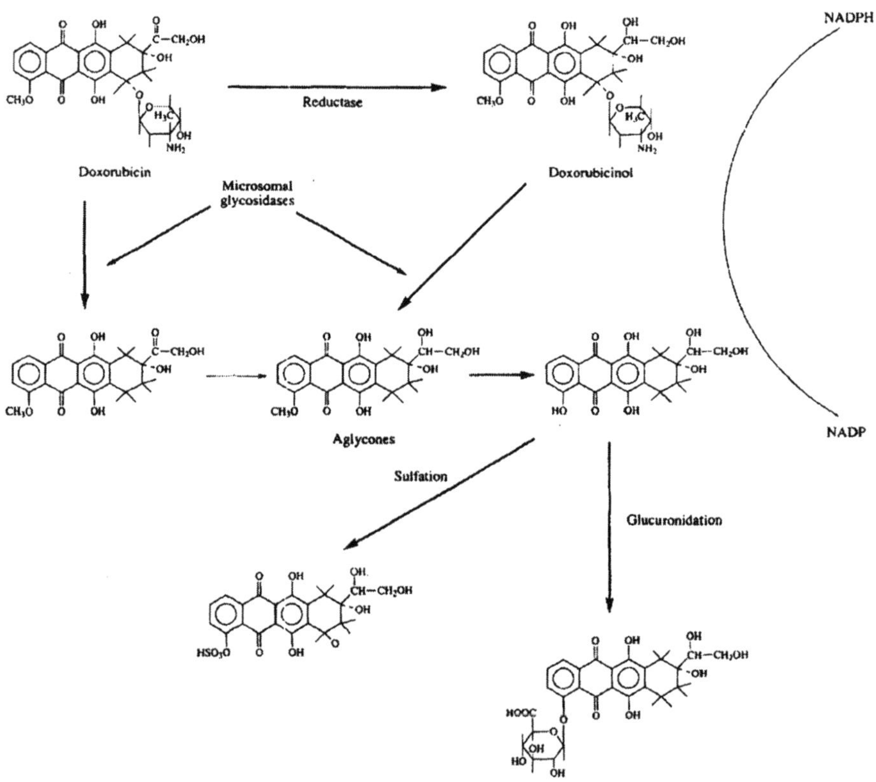

Figure 1 Metabolic pathway of doxorubicin proposed by Bachur[94]

Table 2 Pharmacokinetics of doxorubicin (DOX) in cancer patients with liver dysfunction

Year	*Study/ref.*	*Dose (mg/m^2 i.v.)*	*Diagnosis (no. with liver dysfunction/total)*	*Indices of liver dysfunction (mean value or range)*	*Pharmacokinetic behaviour in the presence of liver dysfunction and authors' comments*
1974	Benjamin et al.[10,11]	60	Disseminated sarcoma (5/8)	Bil > 3 mg/100 ml	Plasma levels of DOX and DOXol 4–5 times higher, delayed drug elimination with severe pancytopenia. 75% dose reduction suggested for bilirubin > 3 mg/100 ml
1980	Chan et al.[15]	15–45	Hepatoma or liver metastases (8/17)	Bil (3–10 × normal, 4 patients), AST (8 × normal), ALT (8 × normal)	Plasma profile of DOX normal, but delayed appearance and prolonged half-life of DOXol in patients with high bilirubin, treated with one-third of the dose
1988	Mross et al.[12]	40–56	Breast cancer with liver metastases (3/8)	γ-GT (> 2 × normal), AST (2–3 × normal), ALT (2–3 × normal)	Delayed DOX elimination, but not clearly related to the degree of liver damage. Reduction of the dose for elevated transaminases does not alter pharmacokinetics as compared to normal patients
1989	Morris et al.[17]	12–44	Extrahepatic tumours (5/15)	APH (mild increase), γ-GT (mild increase)	Plasma profile apparently normal
1992	Johnson et al.[19]		Hepatocellular cancer (16/30)	Bil (2 × normal), AST (2–10 × normal)	AUC for DOX and DOXol increased and directly related to mild alterations of serum bilirubin. Neutropenia, although related to serum bilirubin, does not justify dose adjustment
1992	Piscitelli et al.[18]	45–72	Small cell lung cancer (4/31)	Bil (2–6 × normal), γ-GT (> 10 × normal), APH (> 4 × normal), AST (> 5 × normal)	At 2-fold bilirubin no change in DOX profile, but at 6-fold bilirubin AUC was 3 times higher and terminal half-life significantly prolonged. Marked myelotoxicity associated with liver dysfunction

For abbreviations see Table 1. Bil, bilirubin; AUC, area under the concentration versus time curve.

of DOX and its metabolites were very high in these patients, Benjamin suggested reducing the DOX dose by 50% for patients with serum bilirubin between 2 and 3 mg/100 ml or serum transaminases more than three times normal, by 75% for patients with serum bilirubin >3 mg/100 ml, and withholding treatment in patients with bilirubin > 5 mg/ 100 ml.

Administration of DOX to patients with hepatocellular carcinoma or with liver metastases, with mildly altered transaminase levels but normal bilirubin, results in some delay in elimination[12], reduced clearance and impaired hepatic extraction of the drug[13]. Preiss and associates[14] reported that the elimination rate of DOX correlated with that for antipyrine, which is a marker of liver monooxygenase metabolizing capacity, despite the different elimination mechanisms of the two drugs.

Pharmacokinetic studies by other authors[15–81], using full or reduced DOX doses (15–45 mg/m^2, i.v.) according to the scheme proposed by Benjamin, did not confirm the need for severe dose reduction of DOX in patients with moderate hepatic dysfunction. During treatment with reduced doses of DOX, patients with hepatoma and proven cirrhosis, or with liver metastases and slight elevation of transaminases and bilirubin, had an apparently normal DOX profile. However, formation of the metabolite doxorubicinol (DOXol) was mostly slowed overall in patients with elevated bilirubin, and its half-life was prolonged with an increase in the ratio of DOXol to DOX area under the concentration versus time curve (AUC). These studies did not mention toxicity and therapeutic outcome in relation to pharmacokinetics. The observation by Brenner and associates[16] in acute myelocytic leukaemia (AML) may be noteworthy, although not applicable to solid tumours, as dose-limiting myelotoxicity due to chemotherapy is not a concern in AML. These authors reported that, whereas mildly abnormal liver function tests do not affect DOX clearance and toxicity, overt liver impairment, suggesting a conventional dose reduction, results in lower drug toxicity but also a shorter duration of response and survival. More recent studies[18,19] show that the myelotoxicity of DOX at conventional doses (45–72 mg/m^2) is indeed affected by hepatic dysfunction as measured by serum bilirubin. In patients with hepatocellular carcinoma[19], the degree of toxicity was directly related to serum bilirubin concentration but not to any other liver function test or any pharmacokinetic parameter studied, including AUC or elimination half-life of DOX and DOXol. High bilirubin levels were associated with a higher AUC of the compound and more severe myelosuppression, but there was no evidence of a better response after a full dose of DOX in hyperbilirubinaemic patients. In patients with small cell lung cancer, Piscitelli and associates[18] found a clear relationship between systemic exposure to DOX and DOXol, defined by AUC, and degree of myelosuppression. Patients with high bilirubin (3.7 ± 3.6 mg/100 ml) and clearly abnormal liver function had lower DOX clearance and experienced marked myelotoxicity. These results suggest that, in agreement with previous reports for DOX and other anthracyclines[20–24], there is a significant pharmacodynamic relationship between systemic exposure (AUC) to DOX and myelosuppression. Other DOX-induced toxicities appear to be related to the peak plasma concentration rather than to AUC[25–27], and therefore prolonged infusion schedules have been attempted in order to lower the toxic peak concentrations while maintaining total drug availability[28].

Considering the whole pharmacokinetic literature and the conflicting reports, an indiscriminate dose reduction does not appear to be justified, and may significantly reduce not only toxicity but also the therapeutic outcome. Only for severe liver impairment (i.e. in patients with serum bilirubin > 3 mg/100 ml), is dose adjustment advisable. The AUC of DOX at the first course of therapy may be estimated so as to tailor subsequent doses to each patient, and limited sampling strategies[29] may help to improve drug monitoring.

ANTHRACYCLINE ANALOGUES AND RELATED COMPOUNDS

As far as anthracycline analogues are concerned (Table 3), the association between pharmacokinetics and liver disease has been widely investigated[30–34] for 4′epidoxorubicin (4′epiDOX). In patients with abnormal liver function tests or liver metastases, decreased clearance of 4′epiDOX with delayed plasma elimination of the native compound and of its reduced metabolite, 4′epidoxorubicinol, and increased AUC values of 4′epiDOX, have been reported by the majority of authors. As for DOX, conventional dose reduction of 4′epiDOX based on bilirubin levels has been suggested for clinical practice. These papers, however, give little reliable information about the clinical outcome of treatment. In patients with breast cancer, Speth and associates[31] and Jakobsen and associates[33] described prolonged half-life and reduced clearance of 4′epiDOX in patients with severe hyperbilirubinaemia, as compared with patients with normal liver function.

Based on the finding of a reverse relationship between 4′epiDOX clearance and AST, Twelves and associates[34] suggested that serum AST, rather than serum bilirubin, might be the best indicator of liver impairment and may provide a more rational basis for dose reduction. A rise in AST, reflecting necrosis related to liver involvement by metastases, should arise earlier and precede alterations in bilirubin, which is a less sensitive parameter and reflects serious liver injury. Liver metastases result in an elevated AUC and reduced plasma clearance of 4′epiDOX with increased toxicity[30–35], thus suggesting the need for dose reduction.

In patients with liver dysfunction, 4′epiDOX glucuronidation is affected and the drug total body clearance decreases. Robert and associates[32] observed that patients with reduced hepatic synthesis of several proteins (fibrinogen and globulins) had limited liver glucuronidation capacity with low levels of inactive 4′epiDOX glucuronides and higher availability of the parent compound. These patients had a much lower percentage of change in granulocytes after therapy and responded better to treatment. In this connection the only two patients of Speth's group who achieved partial response had high bilirubin levels with increased concentrations of 4′epiDOX in blood and in haematopoietic cells.

Although the present studies do not permit any firm conclusion on the relationship between impaired liver function, 4′epiDOX pharmacokinetics and pharmacodynamic response, the observations reported do not indicate the need for dose reduction in the presence of mild liver dysfunction, but suggest caution in patients with liver metastases[34]. As observed for DOX by Brenner and associates[16] and by Speth and associates for this DOX analogue[31], higher drug levels may even result in a better response, although at the risk of heavier toxicity.

The pharmacokinetics of the daunomycin analogue, 4-demethoxy daunomycin (idarubicin), have been described by Zanette and associates[36] and by Camaggi and associates[37] in patients with different tumours and liver metastases,

Table 3 Pharmacokinetics of anthracycline analogues and derivatives in cancer patients with liver dysfunction

Year	*Study/ref.*	*Drug and dose (mg/m^2 i.v.)*	*Diagnosis (no. with liver dysfunction/total)*	*Indices of liver dysfunction*	*Pharmacokinetic behaviour in the presence of liver dysfunction and authors' comments*
1992	Camaggi et al.[30]	4-epiDOX (50–90)	Solid tumours with liver metastases (6/17)	Bil, AST, ALT, APH (actual values not reported)	Decreased clearance of epiDOX in two patients, but unchanged pharmacokinetics of epiDOXol. Dose modification suggested in the presence of liver dysfunction
1986	Speth et al.[31]	4-epiDOX (20)	Breast cancer (2/12)	Bil (2–10 × normal)	Decreased clearance and prolonged half-life of epiDOX and epiDOXol, resulting in higher drug levels in white blood cells and improved partial drug response
1991	Jakobsen et al.[33]	4-epiDOX (63)	Breast cancer with liver metastases (3/78)	Bil (3–5 × normal)	Extremely long half-life and increased AUC
1992	Twelves et al.[34]	4-epiDOX (25)	Breast cancer (30/52)	Bil (2–10 × normal), AST (2–5 × normal)	EpiDOX clearance significantly reduced in patients with raised AST. Strong correlation between epiDOX clearance and AST, but not with bilirubin. Serum AST, rather than bilirubin, may be a better indicator for dose adjustment
1990	Zanette et al.[36]	4-DMDR (5) and 5, 10, 25 oral	Different tumours (7/28)	Bil (1.5–2 × normal, 3 patients), γ-GT (2–8 × normal), APH (1.5–6 × normal)	No changes in the kinetics of the drug and its metabolite, 4DMDRol, in the presence of mild liver insufficiency
1992	Camaggi et al.[37]	4-DMDR (12) and 5, 10, 25 oral	Advanced cancer with liver metastases or liver dysfunction (11/21)	AST (1.5–4 × normal), ALT (1.5–8 × normal), APH (1.5–2 × normal)	Kinetics of the drug not significantly influenced
1982	Savaraj et al.[39]	Mitoxantrone (1–12)	Epidermoid cancer of lung and colon (2/11)	Bil (> 2 × normal), AST, APH (actual values not reported)	Decreased clearance and prolonged half-life. Dose modification suggested in liver dysfunction
1986	Smyth et al.[40]	Mitoxantrone (14)	Extrahepatic tumours (2/11 with liver metastases)	Bil (> 2 × normal) γ-GT, APH (actual values not reported)	Prolonged half-life. Dose modification suggested in liver dysfunction

For abbreviations see Tables 1 and 2; 4-DMDR, 4-demethoxydaunorubicin; 4-DMDRol, 4-demethoxydaunorubicinol.

but normal or slightly altered bilirubin levels. Besides a somewhat lower plasma availability of the metabolite, i.e. reduced plasma AUC, no substantial difference was observed compared with patients without liver involvement. Unlike with 4′epiDOX, the pharmacokinetics of idarubicin was not significantly dependent on the presence of liver metastases, but was to some extent related to renal function, since a relationship was found between the clearance of the compound and creatinine[37].

Previous studies reported similar observations in two patients with gastrointestinal carcinoma and extrahepatic biliary obstruction[38] and in patients with different tumours and mild liver impairment[36]. However, although mild liver disease does not seem to require dose modifications, there is too little detailed information on the pharmacokinetic–pharmacodynamic profile in the presence of severe liver dysfunction to establish clear dosing guidelines for 4′epiDOX.

Controversial findings have been reported on the pharmacokinetics of the anthracenedione derivative, mitoxantrone. This compound, which is metabolized and eliminated primarily by the hepatic route, was described by Savaraj and associates[39] and by Smyth and associates[40] as being cleared more slowly, with a prolonged half-life, although not to a remarkable extent, in few cancer patients with apparently moderately abnormal liver function (only bilirubin was reported) or with hepatic metastases. Van Belle and associates[41] found no change in drug kinetics in six patients with liver metastases, even in one with jaundice, but no quantitative data on liver function were provided.

Overall, these findings, together with the observation that no unexpected toxicity was observed in these patients, suggest that dose adjustment is not indispensable in the case of modest liver dysfunction.

ANTIMETABOLITES

Table 4 summarizes the main studies on 5-fluorouracil (5-FU), methotrexate and cyclophosphamide. Hepatic metabolism is the major route of elimination of 5-FU. Christophidis and associates[42] studied 5-FU distribution in 12 patients with colorectal cancer, divided into two groups, with low or high drug availability, but differences in drug bioavailability were not related to differences in liver function or metastatic tumour deposits in the liver. Subsequent studies[43–46] of plasma and tissue concentrations of 5-FU or its derivatives in patients with hepatocellular carcinoma and liver cirrhosis or liver metastases detected no change in drug disposition in relation to liver dysfunction. It would thus seem that no dose adjustment is required for 5-FU and derivatives in this population.

In agreement with an old report[47] of altered drug clearance in patients with hepatic metastases, Port and associates[48] noted a different catabolism of 5-FU in the hepatic tumour tissue in patients with liver metastases from different primary tumours. This finding is difficult to interpret and has limited value on account of the very small number of patients involved.

For methotrexate (MTX), which is mainly excreted through the renal route and whose liver metabolite 7-hydroxymethotrexate is quantitatively irrelevant, hepatic function is not expected to be involved in systemic clearance of the drug. Crom and associates[49] found that abnormal ALT concentrations were associated with lower drug clearance only in patients whose creatinine clearance was near the low limit of the normal range; therefore the liver may play an important role in systemic clearance only for these patients.

The impact of variability in MTX clearance on clinical outcome was clearly documented in children[50,51]. Skoglund and associates[52] found no correlation between drug levels in plasma or urine and liver function tests in children with acute lymphocytic leukaemia and mild liver injury (no liver function test results are given) treated with oral MTX.

CYCLOPHOSPHAMIDE AND RELATED COMPOUNDS

The pharmacokinetic profile of cyclophosphamide (CTX) in patients with liver dysfunction was investigated several years ago by Bagley and associates[53], who reported a prolonged half-life in one patient with cirrhosis and jaundice. Subsequent studies[54,55] in patients with impaired liver function due to metastatic deposits in the liver[54] or to liver cirrhosis due to chronic hepatitis[55] are summarized in Table 4.

Systemic clearance of this compound, which undergoes extensive biotransformation to the active metabolite 4-hydroxy-CTX and then to the inactive 4-keto-CTX and 4-carboxy-CTX in the liver[56] (see Figure 2) should be influenced by liver function. However, in patients with moderate liver dysfunction, indicated by changes in pseudocholinesterase serum levels, reduced clearance and prolonged half-life of CTX, and the delayed appearance and inactivation of 4-hydroxy-CTX, overall exposure to the active metabolites does not change. In agreement with this pharmacokinetic finding, Juma[55] observed no clinical evidence of increased toxicity even in patients with severely affected liver function, so apparently no dosage adjustment is needed in the presence of liver disease.

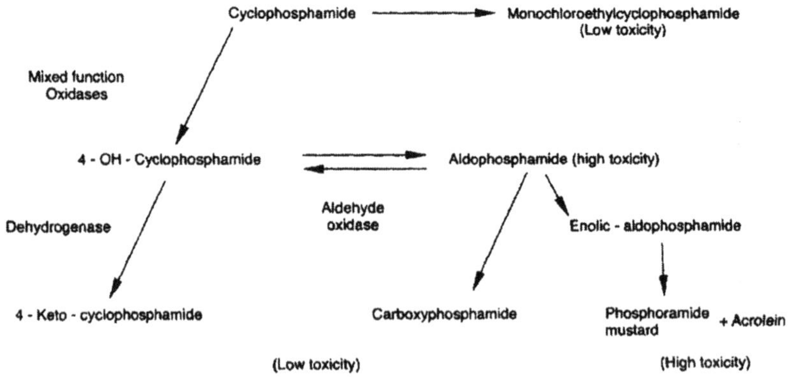

Figure 2 Metabolic pathway of cyclophosphamide modified; by permission of *Biochemical Pharmacology*[95]

Table 4 Pharmacokinetics of 5-fluorouracil (5-FU), methotrexate (MTX) and cyclophosphamide (CTX) in cancer patients with liver dysfunction

Year	*Study/ref.*	*Drug and dose (mg/m^2)*	*Diagnosis (no. with liver dysfunction/total)*	*Indices of liver dysfunction*	*Pharmacokinetic behaviour in the presence of liver dysfunction and authors' comments*
1992	Fleming et al.[46]	5-FU (552–1069 i.v.)	Head and neck cancer (187 patients, with and without liver dysfunction)	Bil, AST, ALT, APH, γ-GT (actual values not reported)	A poor linear correlation ($p < 0.05$) between drug clearance and liver dysfunction values was found only for APH, but not for the other liver tests. No dose reduction is indicated
1994	Skoglund et al.[52]	MTX (4–29 per os)	ALL and non-Hodgkin's lymphoma (15/17)	Bil, AST, ALT, APH, γ-GT (mild alterations, but actual values not reported)	No correlation was found between serum levels of MTX or its 7-OH metabolite and liver function tests
1980	Von Wagner et al.[54]	CTX (10 i.v.)	Metastatic carcinoma (10/20 with liver metastases)	CHE (< 3000 U/L)	Reduced clearance of native drug and lower serum levels of activated CTX. However, due to low renal clearance, AUC of CTX metabolites remains relatively unchanged
1984	Juma[55]	CTX (15 i.v.)	Hodgkin disease (7/17 with liver cirrhosis)	Bil (7 × normal), AST (9 × normal), ALT (6 × normal), APH (8 × normal)	These patients with severe liver injury have a longer half-life and lower total body clearance of the native compound. No evidence of increased toxicity

For abbreviations see Tables 1 and 2; ALL, acute lymphocytic leukaemia.

Table 5 Pharmacokinetics of vincristine in cancer patients with liver dysfunction

Year	*Study/ref.*	*Dose (mg/m^2 i.v.)*	*Diagnosis (no. with liver dysfunction/total)*	*Indices of liver dysfunction*	*Pharmacokinetic behaviour in the presence of liver dysfunction and authors' comments*
1992	Van den Berg[60]	0.4–1.5	Different tumours (15/39)	Bil (3 patients), AST, ALT, APH, γ-GT (actual values not reported)	Prolonged β half-life and higher plasma AUC account for reduced clearance in the presence of cholestasis
1992	Desai et al.[61]	1.4–2	Leukaemia and lymphoma (11/27)	APH (83% increase in 5 patients)	Significant correlation between dose, AUC and neuropathy. Higher plasma AUC accounts for impaired drug elimination. Increased toxicity in patients with high APH suggests dose reduction, even with normal bilirubin and transaminases

For abbreviations see Tables 1 and 2; ALL, acute lymphocytic leukaemia.

It is reasonable to assume that the same conclusions should apply to the CTX derivative, iphosphamide, which undergoes the same metabolic transformation, but whose pharmacokinetics in the presence of liver impairment has, to our knowledge, not been described.

VINCA ALKALOIDS AND TAXANES

The tubulin acting agents are the only clear example (Table 5) of antitumour agents requiring dose adjustment in cancer patients with liver dysfunction: vincristine, vinblastine, apparently vinorelbine and the taxane compounds, paclitaxel and docetaxel.

A consistent finding in clinical trials after repeated doses of vincristine (VCR) is neurotoxicity, which is related to the cumulative dose[57]. As the biliary system is the main route of excretion of VCR and its desacetyl-metabolic products[58], it is reasonable to expect that, in spite of significant individual differences in the pharmacokinetics of VCR[59], hepatic dysfunction and especially cholestasis might alter elimination kinetics and increase exposure to the drug and its metabolites, thus increasing toxicity.

Van den Berg and associates[60] and Desai and associates[61] investigated the pharmacokinetic behaviour of VCR in patients with different tumours and cholestasis, with increased serum levels of alkaline phosphatase and, in several cases, also bilirubin. In patients with liver dysfunction the half-life of VCR is more than doubled and the total availability, expressed by the AUC, is three times higher than in patients with normal liver function. Neurotoxicity was related to the dose and to the plasma AUC of the drug. Desai and associates[61] noted that, in cholestatic patients, a small reduction in the drug dose resulted in lower VCR plasma AUC and less neurotoxicity. They did not indicate the extent to which alkaline phosphatase (APH) or bilirubin was raised in these patients. However, in view of the clinical evidence of toxicity, it is reasonable to recommend dose adjustment in the presence of cholestasis.

Similar considerations apply to the VCR-related compound, vinblastine (VBL). Although a decrease in drug clearance seems related to the response rate[62], in patients who have received prolonged drug infusions high serum drug concentrations are only weakly associated with the severe leucopenia resulting from treatment, but strongly related to non-haematological toxicity[63]. These observations suggest that a dose reduction should also be considered in patients with liver dysfunction receiving this drug.

The new semisynthetic vinca alkaloid, vinorelbine, has been investigated in advanced breast cancer patients with liver metastases[64]. In patients with severe liver dysfunction, indicated by the dynamic mono-ethylglycine-xylidide test (MEGX) for formation of the lidocaine metabolite, and by bilirubin and AST, drug clearance is markedly reduced and significantly correlated only with MEGX and bilirubin. For vinorelbine, therefore, as for the other vinca alkaloids, dose reduction is recommended in patients with severe liver dysfunction, but not those with moderate liver involvement.

Taxanes, which enhance microtubule assembly and inhibit tubulin depolymerization[65], are metabolized mainly through the liver and undergo biliary

Table 6 Pharmacokinetics of etoposide in cancer patients with liver dysfunction

Year	*Study/ref.*	*Dose (mg/m^2 i.v.)*	*Diagnosis (no. with liver dysfunction/total)*	*Indices of liver dysfunction*	*Pharmacokinetic behaviour*	*Authors' comments*
1986	Arbruck et al.[81]	100 × 3	Different carcinomas (8/17 hepatobiliary tumours)	Bil (2–10 × normal), AST (2 × normal), APH (2–5 × normal)	Cls (ml/min/m^2): 21.4 + 7.4 in C, 22.4 + 9.6 in Ld $\beta_{t1/2}$ (h): 8.1 + 2.8 in C, 8.4 + 3.9 in Ld	No changes in etoposide kinetics in the presence of liver dysfunction. Dose reduction may not be required
1986	D'Incalci et al.[82]	80–150 × 1 or 3	Hepatocarcinoma or extrahepatic tumours with/without liver metastases (15/33)	Bil (2–20 × normal, 9 patients), γ-GT (3–20 × normal), APH (2–7 × normal)	Cls (ml/min/m^2): 22.8 + 1.0 in C, 27.9+2.7 in Ld $\beta_{t1/2}$ (h): 5.6 + 0.4 in C, 5.4 + 0.6 in Ld	No changes in etoposide kinetics in the presence of liver dysfunction. However, in three patients with severe cholestasis clearance was low (> 87 ml/min/m^2). Dose reduction may not be required except in presence of cholestasis
1990	Hande et al.[83]	100–800	Obstructive jaundice in patients with cancer (11/33)	Bil (2–12 × normal), AST (3–6 × normal), APH (28 × normal)	Cls (ml/min/m^2): 26.5 + 9.5 in C, 24.5 + 6.5 in Ld $\beta_{t1/2}$ (h): 6.4 + 2.5 in C, 5.7 + 1.5 in Ld	No changes in etoposide kinetics in the presence of liver dysfunction. Standard doses should be used in patients with obstructive biliary disease
1996	Joel et al.[84]	500	Small cell lung cancer (total 72 patients)	AST or γ-GT with albumin ≥ 35 g/L, mild (1.5–3 × normal, 3 patients) severe (> 3 × normal, 4 patients), albumin < 35 g/L	AUC (μg/ml × h) total 457, free 16.6; total 536, free 20.2; total 425, free 22.8; total 463, free 27.4	No changes in the kinetics of total etoposide in the presence of liver dysfunction. However, severe liver dysfunction, even more with low albumin levels, results in an increase of the free drug and more pronounced haematological toxicity. Dose reduction is advisable in patients with low albumin
1995	Liu et al.[85]	50 mg/day oral or i.v.	Different solid tumours and two lymphomas	Bil (2–10 × normal, 6 patients), APH (1.5–12 × normal), albumin (< 30 g/L, 12 patients)		Free fraction of etoposide shows a strong negative correlation with serum albumin ($p < 0.0001$), but not with serum bilirubin

See legends to Tables 1 and 2.
C, controls; Ld, liver dysfunction; Cls, systemic clearance; $\beta_{t1/2}$, β half-life.

excretion[66]. Two main metabolites of paclitaxel, corresponding to hydroxylation at the C6 position of the taxane ring and at the para position of the phenyl ring at the C3 position of the C13 side chain, account for 70% of biliary excretion. A retrospective finding from preliminary reports by Egorin and associates[67] and Venook and associates[68] suggests that in patients with severely affected liver function (bilirubin higher than 3 mg/100 ml), the serum concentration of paclitaxel at the steady state is higher and the total body clearance after 24-h infusion lower than in patients with normal bilirubin.

Dose-limiting toxicity, mostly neutropenia, was observed in patients with high bilirubin levels. Similar results were obtained by Wilson and associates[69] in a phase II study with a 96-h infusion of paclitaxel in patients with liver metastases but bilirubin not higher than 2 mg/100 ml. Metastatic liver disease was strongly associated with reduced drug clearance, higher steady-state concentrations and increased haematological toxicity. The extent of liver involvement, evaluated by computed tomography, was inversely correlated with paclitaxel clearance. Therefore it was suggested that, in patients with evidence of extensive liver metastases or liver disease with clearly abnormal liver function tests, the starting dose of paclitaxel should be reduced by 30%. This same report noted that serum levels of AST were significantly related to the presence of liver metastases. Therefore, the authors suggested that AST may be a better predictor of liver dysfunction and of decreased drug clearance than total bilirubin, which was not substantially altered in these patients. Seidman and associates[70] reduced the dose, which proved to be safe in metastatic breast cancer patients with hepatic dysfunction, as reflected by elevation of AST and ALT more than twice the upper limit of normal. The steady-state concentration of paclitaxel, which was twice as high as in patients with normal transaminases, was directly related to the incidence of grade 4 neutropenia, but there was no relationship between serum drug levels and response. However, further studies with a prospective design are clearly required.

As regards the neurotoxicity of paclitaxel, it is dosage-schedule dependent[71] and roughly correlates with the AUC[72]. However, appropriate clinical trials relating drug-induced neuropathy and pharmacokinetic parameters are not yet available.

The semisynthetic taxane analogue docetaxel has been investigated extensively in phase I and II population pharmacokinetic studies[73]. Although Bruno and associates[74] reported that drug clearance was correlated with plasma hepatic enzyme levels, in patients with 'elevated hepatic enzymes' a 30% reduction in clearance did not seem to modify significantly the toxic or therapeutic response. Hudis and associates[75] confirmed in 34 patients that the total drug availability as expressed by the AUC did not apparently correlate with toxicity. However, in this study one patient with hepatic metastases and pretreatment bilirubin of 1.8 mg/100 ml, resulting in a much higher steady-state level (11.6 μg/ml versus a median of 4.6 μg/ml for the other patients) and decreased docetaxel clearance, died with extensive haematological and non-haematological toxicity.

That the risk of toxicity (neutropenia and mucositis) with docetaxel increases with liver metastases and elevated AST and alkaline phosphatase serum levels has been previously observed[76]. Therefore, caution is warranted and dose reduction seems advisable for docetaxel when treating patients with liver dysfunction, although the correlation between pharmacokinetic parameters and toxicity needs further investigation.

EPIPODOPHYLLOTOXINS

The epipodophyllotoxins etoposide (VP16) and teniposide (VM26) are widely used antitumour compounds, whose pharmacokinetics in the presence of organ failure has been investigated. VP16 and VM26 in humans are cleared both by the kidneys and by direct hepatobiliary metabolism and excretion of the inactive glucuronide and sulphate derivatives[77]. Impairment of liver function may reduce the rate of metabolism and/or biliary excretion of these compounds, thus increasing toxicity. Therefore, in clinical practice in patients with elevated bilirubin the dose is often reduced. Dose reduction, however, may compromise achievement of the drug serum concentrations needed for optimal response to therapy. Slevin and associates[78] demonstrated that the therapeutic effect of etoposide is related to the presence of a critical drug level for a given time. Rodman and associates[79] established a similar relationship for VM26, showing good correlation between drug steady-state concentration or clearance and response rate in children.

Several studies are available on the pharmacokinetics of VP16 and VM26, administered intravenously to patients with primary or metastatic liver cancer or with liver dysfunction of different origin. Sinkule and associates[80] suggested that the decreased clearance and prolonged half-life of VP16 in four children with high serum transaminases might be attributable to the concomitant lower creatinine clearance induced by prior cisplatin treatment. Results of other studies are summarized in Table 6, with the pharmacokinetic parameters for comparison. Arbruck and associates[81], D'Incalci and associates[82] and Hande and associates[83] found neither decreased total body clearance nor prolonged half-life of total VP16 in patients with severe liver dysfunction (bilirubin often ten times normal) even when associated with obstructive jaundice, as the low liver metabolic clearance in these patients is compensated by an increase in renal clearance. Meta-analysis of the combined data[83] clearly indicates that the serum pharmacokinetics of the total drug is not significantly altered in the presence of liver impairment.

On the basis of the information outlined in these pharmacokinetic studies, normal intravenous doses of VP16 should be given to patients with liver dysfunction. However, caution should be used in patients with severe liver dysfunction and renal impairment, in whom the decrease in metabolic clearance cannot be compensated by increased renal clearance.

Alternatively, an increased fraction of the unbound active drug directly related to high serum bilirubin and low albumin levels might explain the increased pharmacological and toxic effects (neutropenia) of standard VP16 doses in patients with liver disease[84]. Other authors[85], while confirming this finding for albumin, were not able to demonstrate a clear relationship between serum bilirubin levels and protein binding. Similar pharmacokinetic behaviour was reported for prolonged oral treatment with VP16[86,87]. The consideration that severe neutropenia may occur after prolonged oral treatment suggests that, apart from any pharmacokinetic consideration, it may be advisable to monitor neutrophil count often during oral VP16 treatment in patients with liver dysfunction.

Two papers describe the pharmacokinetics of the VP16 analogue, VM26[88,89]. In children with leukaemia, Canal and associates reported a significant inverse relationship between APH and systemic clearance of VM26, while in patients with ovarian carcinoma an inverse correlation was found between γ-GT and plasma clearance of the compound. However, these data come from small groups of patients whose clearance was only moderately reduced and, although they emphasize the role of the liver in drug clearance, they are not sufficient to establish dosage guidelines.

DISCUSSION

This review looks at the pharmacokinetics of selected anticancer agents in the presence of liver impairment. The aim was to assess whether guidelines for dose adjustments could be extrapolated from pharmacokinetic studies, but the conclusion is that in most instances the empirical dose adjustments that are still the rule in clinical practice are not justified by experimental data.

Conventional doses of anticancer drugs are established by phase 1 trials to fit the balance between optimal therapeutic effects and safety in the average population of patients. The need for dose adjustment is based on the recognition that individual patients may be different from 'normal' patients, so that standard doses may have lower efficacy or worse toxicity than expected. Patients with liver dysfunction clearly deviate from the norm in many ways, such as their total body clearance and disposition, that may affect key pharmacokinetic parameters of anticancer drugs and the pharmacodynamic consequences of their administration.

It would appear obvious that dose adjustments must be tailored on the basis of established relationships between specific indices of liver dysfunction and the ensuing pharmacokinetic alterations. However, guidelines are lacking since their definition depends both on the type and extent of liver disease, and on the unique characteristics of each drug. Guidelines can be established only by studying homogeneous patient populations in terms of diagnosis and by stratifying patients according to the severity of liver disease. However, these key criteria were not met in almost all the studies reviewed.

The case of the anthracyclines is typical in this respect[90]. In spite of years of technically adequate measurements of anthracycline pharmacokinetics, data were collected from patients in whom abnormal liver biochemistry was associated with different liver diseases, such as metastases, primary liver cancer or non-neoplastic liver diseases of different aetiologies. Therefore, different studies often reported conflicting results. As a result the dose of doxorubicin or epirubicin is still empirically adjusted, on the basis of serum bilirubin.

For the other major antineoplastic agents the information available in the literature indicates that in patients with moderate liver dysfunction their clearance does not appear to be substantially modified. Therefore, dose reduction is not necessarily recommended, since it could lead to ineffective therapeutic levels. In fact, although caution is compulsory in treating patients with impaired organ function, considerations of the risks of toxicity should not compromise the achievement of therapeutic benefit.

For the vinca alkaloids, VCR, VLB and vinorelbine, there is strong evidence that dose reduction is mandatory in the presence of liver impairment, particularly severe impairment, and especially with cholestasis. Dose adjustment seems to be advisable also for the newer compounds paclitaxel and docetaxel, which are cleared more slowly in patients with elevated bilirubin[67,68,75] or other liver enzymes such as AST and APH[69,74,76]. However, at present, only a reduction in clearance appears to be directly correlated with increased haematological toxicity and mucositis[70,76] and no relationship has been found between serum drug levels and response[70,74,75].

A clinically important question is whether biochemical indices of liver dysfunction predict alterations in drug clearance. To our knowledge the only reports dealing with this are by Twelves and associates for epirubicin[34] and Wilson and associates[69] for paclitaxel. Evidence was provided that serum levels of AST, a good predictor of survival in cancer patients with liver metastases[91], may provide a more rational basis for dose adjustment in cancer patients treated with epirubicin or paclitaxel than the currently recommended bilirubin, which does not always show appreciable changes.

The same considerations may possibly apply to docetaxel[76], although the limited number and broad heterogeneity of the patients studied, as well as the uneven characterization of the aetiology and severity of liver disease, do not permit any general conclusion. However, there is an interesting relationship between the extent of liver involvement and paclitaxel clearance in patients with metastatic breast cancer[69]. For patients with primary or secondary liver cancer it would be useful to establish a relationship between the size of the tumour, which is easily measured by ultrasonography, and the changes in pharmacokinetic parameters. Studies specifically aimed at establishing such relationships are warranted, at least for drugs whose pharmacokinetics change in the presence of liver dysfunction. Various biochemical indices of liver impairment that might predict changes in drug pharmacokinetics should be further investigated. Parameters of liver dysfunction may be related to necrosis and inflammation (AST and ALT), to cholestasis (total and esterified bilirubin, bile acids, albumin, γ-GT), or to reduced hepatocellular mass leading to impairment of liver function (mainly the quantitative dynamic tests, such as those based on antipyrine or lidocaine metabolite formation or on galactose elimination capacity). Among the dynamic tests the relatively new MEGX test correlates with the liver histological status better than the other biochemical tests[64] and has some prognostic significance, as low MEGX levels were limited to poor survival[92].

To design specific studies aimed at establishing guidelines for dose adjustment of antineoplastic agents in patients with liver diseases, the type and degree of liver dysfunction must be clearly defined. Moreover, as severe liver disease is often associated with other structural and functional organ abnormalities such as renal impairment, the patients' general pathophysiological state must always be checked.

In conclusion, liver dysfunction is often associated with abnormal clearance of anticancer agents. Dose adjustment according to pharmacokinetic guidelines is needed in order to avoid the risk of undertreatment often associated with empirical criteria. Future clinical studies might assess relationships between markers of liver disease, disposition of anticancer agents and their safety in groups of patients homogeneous for aetiology and stratified for the degree of liver impairment.

Acknowledgements

The authors thank Vanna Pisotti of the Gustavus A. Pfeiffer Memorial Library for much help in collecting the bibliography through a Medline search. This work was supported in part by the Italian Association for Cancer Research and by funds of the Ministry of Scientific Research (MURST 60%).

References

1. Stewart CF, Pieper JA, Arbuck SG et al. Altered protein binding of etoposide in patients with cancer. Clin Pharmacol Ther. 1989;45:49–55.
2. Pfluger KH, Schmidt L, Merkel M et al. Drug monitoring of etoposide (VP16–213). Correlation of pharmacokinetic parameters to clinical and biochemical data from patients receiving etoposide. Cancer Chemother Pharmacol. 1987;20:59–66.
3. Ratain MJ, Vogelzang NJ, Sinkule JA. Interpatient and intrapatient variability in vinblastine pharmacokinetics. Clin Pharmacol Ther. 1987;41:61–7.
4. Powis G. Effect of human renal and hepatic disease on the pharmacokinetics of anticancer drugs. Cancer Treat Rev. 1982;9:85–124.
5. Koren G, Beatty K, Seto A et al. The effects of impaired liver function on the elimination of antineoplastic agents. Ann Pharmacother. 1992;26:363–71.
6. Muraca M, Fevery J, Blanckaert N. Analytic aspects and clinical interpretation of serum bilirubins. Semin Liver Dis. 1988;8:137–47.
7. Shiffman ML, Luketic VA, Sanyal AJ et al. Hepatic lidocaine metabolism and liver histology in patients with chronic hepatitis and cirrhosis. Hepatology. 1994;19:933–40.
8. Pritchard-Davies R, Gross AS, Shenfield GM. The effect of liver disease and food on plasma MEGX concentrations. Br J Clin Pharmacol. 1994;37:298–301.
9. August DA, Halter S, Brenner DE. Effect of sublethal liver injury on doxorubicin metabolism. Clin Cancer Res. 1995;1:351–8.
10. Benjamin RS, Wiernik PH, Bachur NR. Adriamycin chemotherapy – efficacy, safety, and pharmacologic basis of an intermittent single high-dosage schedule. Cancer. 1974;33:19–27.
11. Benjamin RS. Pharmacokinetics of adriamycin (NSC-123127) in patients with sarcomas. Cancer Chemother Rep. 1974;58:271–3.
12. Mross K, Maessen P, van der Vijgh WJF et al. Pharmacokinetics and metabolism of epidoxorubicin and doxorubicin in humans. Clin Oncol. 1988;6:517–26.
13. Ballet F, Barbare JC, Poupon R. Hepatic extraction of adriamycin in patients with hepatocellular carcinoma. Eur Cancer Clin Oncol. 1984;20:761–4.
14. Preiss R, Matthias M, Sohr R et al. Pharmacokinetics of adriamycin, adriamycinol, and antipyrine in patients with moderate tumour involvement of the liver. Cancer Res Clin Oncol. 1987;113:593–8.
15. Chan KK, Chlebowski RT, Tong M et al. Clinical pharmacokinetics of adriamycin in hepatoma patients with cirrhosis. Cancer Res. 1980;40:1263–8.
16. Brenner DE, Wiernik PH, Wesley M et al. Acute doxorubicin toxicity. Relationship to pretreatment liver function, response, and pharmacokinetics in patients with acute nonlymphocytic leukemia. Cancer. 1984;53:1042–8.
17. Morris RG, Reece PA, Dale BM et al. Alteration in doxorubicin and doxorubicinol plasma concentrations with repeated courses to patients. Ther Drug Monit. 1989;11:380–3.
18. Piscitelli SC, Rodvold KA, Rushing DA et al. Pharmacokinetics and pharmacodynamics of doxorubicin in patients with small cell lung cancer. Clin Pharmacol Ther. 1993;53:555–61.
19. Johnson PJ, Dobbs N, Kalayci C et al. Clinical efficacy and toxicity of standard dose adriamycin in hyperbilirubinaemic patients with hepatocellular carcinoma: relation to liver tests and pharmacokinetic parameters. Br J Cancer. 1992;64:751–5.
20. Jakobsen P, Basthop L, Dalmark M et al. A randomized study of epirubicin at four different dose levels in advanced breast cancer. Feasibility of myelotoxicity prediction through single blood sample measurement. Cancer Chemother Pharmacol. 1991;28:465–9.
21. Robert J, Monnier A, Poutignat N et al. A pharmacokinetic and pharmacodynamic study of the new anthracycline pirarubicin in breast cancer patients. Cancer Chemother Pharmacol. 1991;29:75–9.
22. Canal P, Robert J, Ramon M et al. Human pharmacokinetics of N-1-leucildoxorubicin, a new anthracycline derivative, and its correlation with clinical toxicities. Clin Pharmacol Ther. 1992;51:249–59.
23. Elbaek K, Ebbehoy E, Jakobsen A et al. Pharmacokinetics of oral idarubicin in breast cancer patients with reference to antitumor activity and side effects. Clin Pharmacol Ther. 1989;45:627–34.

24. Ackland SP, Ratain MJ, Vogelzang NJ et al. Pharmacokinetics and pharmacodynamics of long-term continuous-infusion doxorubicin. Clin Pharmacol Ther. 1989;45:340–7.
25. Legha SS, Benjamin RS, Mackay B et al. Reduction of doxorubicin cardiotoxicity by prolonged continuous intravenous infusion. Ann Intern Med. 1982;96:133–9.
26. Zalupski M, Metch B, Balcerzak S et al. Phase III comparison of doxorubicin and dacarbazine given by bolus versus infusion in patients with soft-tissue sarcomas: a Southwest Oncology Group Study. J Natl Cancer Inst. 1991;83:926–32.
27. Hortobagyi GN, Frye D, Buzdar AU et al. Decreased cardiac toxicity of doxorubicin administered by continuous intravenous infusion in combination chemotherapy for metastatic breast carcinoma. Cancer. 1989;63:37–45.
28. Workman P. Infusional antracyclines: is slower better? If so, why? Ann Oncol. 1992;3:591–4.
29. Ratain MJ, Robert J, van der Vijgh WJ. Limited sampling models for doxorubicin pharmacokinetics. J Clin Oncol. 1991;9:871–6.
30. Camaggi CM, Strocchi E, Tamassia V et al. Pharmacokinetic studies of 4epi-doxorubicin in cancer patients with normal and impaired renal function and with hepatic metastases. Cancer Treat Rep. 1982;66:1819–24.
31. Speth PAJ, Linssen PCM, Beex LVAM et al. Cellular and plasma pharmacokinetics of weekly 20 mg 4′-epi-adriamycin bolus injection in patients with advanced breast carcinoma. Cancer Chemother Pharmacol. 1986;18:78–82.
32. Robert J, David M, Granger C. Metabolism of epirubicin to glucuronides: relationship to the pharmacodynamics of the drugs. Cancer Chemother Pharmacol. 1990;27:147–50.
33. Jakobsen P, Steiness E, Bastholt L et al. Multiple-dose pharmacokinetics of epirubicin at four different dose levels: studies in patients with metastatic breast cancer. Cancer Chemother Pharmacol. 1991;28:63–8.
34. Twelves C, Dobbs NA, Michael Y et al. Clinical pharmacokinetics of epirubicin: the importance of liver biochemistry tests. Br J Cancer. 1992;66:765–9.
35. Camaggi CM, Comparsi R, Strocchi E et al. Epirubicin and doxorubicin comparative metabolism and pharmacokinetics. A cross-over study. Cancer Chemother Pharmacol. 1988;21:221–8.
36. Zanette L, Zucchetti M, Freschi A et al. Pharmacokinetics of 4demethoxydaunorubicin in cancer patients. Cancer Chemother Pharmacol. 1990;25:445–8.
37. Camaggi CM, Strocchi E, Carisi P et al. Idarubicin metabolism and pharmacokinetics after intravenous and oral administration in cancer patients: a crossover study. Cancer Chemother Pharmacol. 1992;30:307–16.
38. Pannuti F, Camaggi CM, Strocchi E et al. Low dose oral administration of 4demethoxy-daunorubicin (idarubicin) in advanced cancer patients. A pharmacokinetic study. Cancer Chemother Pharmacol. 1986;16:295–9.
39. Savaraj N, Lu K, Manuel V et al. Pharmacology of mitoxantrone in cancer patients. Cancer Chemother Pharmacol. 1982;8:113–17.
40. Smyth JF, Macpherson JS, Warrington PS et al. The clinical pharmacology of mitoxantrone. Cancer Chemother Pharmacol. 1986;17:149–52.
41. Van Belle SJP, de Planque MM, Smith LE et al. Pharmacokinetics of mitoxantrone in humans following single-agent infusion or intra-arterial injection therapy or combined-agent infusion therapy. Cancer Chemother Pharmacol. 1986;18:27–32.
42. Christophidis N, Vajda FJE, Lucas I et al. Fluorouracil therapy in patients with carcinoma of the large bowel: a pharmacokinetic comparison of various rates and routes of administration. Clin Pharmacokinet. 1978;3:330–6.
43. Kawata S, Noda S, Imai Y et al. Hepatic conversion of 1-(tetrahydro-2furanil)-5-fluorouracil into 5-fluorouracil in patients with hepatocellular carcinoma. Gastroententerol Jpn. 1987;22:55–62.
44. Suenaga M. 5-FU and HCFU concentrations in serum and tissues in hepatocellular carcinoma after HCFU oral administration. Gan No Rinsho. 1988;34:744–8.
45. Nowakowska-Dulawa E. Circadian rhythm of 5-fluorouracil (FU) pharmacokinetics and tolerance. Chronologie. 1990;17:27–35.
46. Fleming RA, Milano GA, Etienne MC et al. No effect of dose, hepatic function or nutritional status on 5-FU clearance following continuous (5-day), 5-FU infusion. Br J Cancer. 1992;66:668–72.
47. Floyd RA, Hornbeck CL, Byfield JE et al. Clearance of continuously infused 5-fluorouracil in adults having lung or gastrointestinal carcinoma with or without hepatic metastases. Drug Intell Clin Pharm. 1982;16:665–7.

48. Port RE, Bachen P, Semmler W. Kinetic modeling of in vivo nuclear magnetic resonance spectroscopy data: 5-fluorouracil in liver and liver tumors. Clin Pharmacol Ther. 1991;49:497–505.
49. Crom WR, Glynn AM, Abromowitch M et al. Use of the automatic interaction detector method to identify patient characteristics related to methotrexate clearance. Clin Pharmacol Ther. 1986;39:592–7.
50. Evans WE, Crom WR, Stewart CF et al. Methotrexate systemic clearance influences probability of relapse in children with standard-risk acute lymphocytic leukemia. Lancet. 1984;1:359–62.
51. Evans WE, Crom WR, Abromowitch M et al. Clinical pharmacodynamics of high-dose methotrexate in acute lymphocytic leukemia. N Engl J Med. 1986;314:471–7.
52. Skoglund KA, Soderhall S, Beck O et al. Plasma and urine levels of methotrexate and 7-hydroxymethotrexate in children with ALL during maintenance therapy with weekly oral methotrexate. Med Pediatr Oncol. 1994;22:187–93.
53. Bagley CM Jr, Bostick FW, DeVita VT Jr. Clinical pharmacology of cyclophosphamide. Cancer Res. 1973;33:226–33.
54. Von Wagner T, Heydrich D, Bartels H et al. Einfluss von Leberparenchymschäden, Niereninsuffizienz und Himodialyse auf die Pharmakokinetik von Cyclophosphamid und seiner Aktivierten Metaboliten. Arzneimittelforschung. 1980;30:1588–92.
55. Juma FD. Effect of liver failure on the pharmacokinetics of cyclophosphamide. Eur J Clin Pharmacol. 1984;26:591–3.
56. Fenselau C, Kan MN, Rao SS et al. Identification of aldophosphamide as a metabolite of cyclophosphamide *in vitro* and *in vivo* in humans. Cancer Res. 1977;37:2538–43.
57. Rosenthal S, Kauffman S. Vincristine neurotoxicity. Ann Intern Med. 1974;80:733–7.
58. Jackson DV Jr, Castle MC, Bender RA. Biliary excretion of vincristine. Clin Pharmacol Ther. 1978;24:101–7.
59. Sethi VS, Jackson DV Jr, White DR et al. Pharmacokinetics of vincristine sulfate in adult cancer patients. Cancer Res. 1981;41:3551–5.
60. Van den Berg HW, Desai ZR, Wilson R et al. The pharmacokinetics of vincristine in man: reduced drug clearance associated with raised serum alkaline phosphatase and dose-limited elimination. Cancer Chemother Pharmacol. 1982;8:215–19.
61. Desai ZR, Van den Berg HW, Bridges JM et al. Can severe vincristine neurotoxicity be prevented? Cancer Chemother Pharmacol. 1982;8:211–14.
62. Lu K, Yap HY, Loo TL. Clinical pharmacokinetics of vinblastine by continuous intravenous infusion. Cancer Res. 1983;43:1405–8.
63. Chong CDK, Logothetis C, Savaraj N et al. The correlation of vinblastine pharmacokinetics to toxicity in testicular cancer patients. J Clin Pharmacol. 1988;28:714–18.
64. Robieux I, Sorio R, Borsatti E et al. Pharmacokinetics of vinorelbine in patients with liver metastases. Clin Pharmacol Ther. 1996;59:32–40.
65. Gueritte-Voegelein F, Guenard D, Lavelle F et al. Relationships between the structure of Taxol analogues and their antimitotic activity. J Med Chem. 1991;34:992–8.
66. Cresteil T, Monsarrat B, Alvinerie P et al. Taxol metabolism by human liver microsomes: Identification of cytochrome P450 isozymes involved in its biotransformation. Cancer Res. 1994;54:386–92.
67. Egorin M, Venook A, Jahan T et al. Plasma pharmacokinetics and biliary excretion of paclitaxel in patients with hepatic dysfunction. Ann Oncol. 1994;5(Suppl. 5):196.
68. Venook AP, Egorin M, Brown TD et al. Paclitaxel (Taxol) in patients with liver dysfunction (CALGB 9264). Proc Am Soc Clin Oncol. 1994;13:139.
69. Wilson WH, Berg SL, Bryant G et al. Paclitaxel in doxorubicin-refractory or mitoxantrone-refractory breast cancer: a phase I/II trial of 96-hour infusion. J Clin Oncol. 1984;12:1621–9.
70. Seidman AD, Hochhauser D, Gollub M et al. Ninety-six-hour paclitaxel infusion after progression during short taxane exposure: a phase II pharmacokinetic and pharmacodynamic study in metastatic breast cancer. J Clin Oncol. 1996;14:1877–84.
71. Vermorken JB, Postma TJ, Pinedo HM et al. Neuropathic symptoms and signs with 3-hour paclitaxel. Ann Oncol. 1994;5(Suppl. 5):196.
72. Brown T, Havlin K, Weiss G et al. A phase I trial of taxol given by 6-hour intravenous infusion. J Clin Oncol. 1991;9:1261–7.
73. Launay-Iliadis MC, Bruno R, Cosson V et al. Population pharmacokinetics of docetaxel during phase I studies using nonlinear mixed-effect modeling and nonparametric maximum-likelihood estimation. Cancer Chemother Pharmacol. 1995;37:47–54.

74. Bruno R, Hille D, Thomas L, Riva A, Sheiner LB. Population pharmacokinetics/pharmacodynamics (PK/PD) of docetaxel (Taxoterel®) in phase II studies. Proc Am Soc Clin Oncol. 1995;14:457.
75. Hudis CA, Seidman AD, Crown JPA et al. Phase II and pharmacologic study of docetaxel as initial chemotherapy for metastatic breast cancer. J Clin Oncol. 1996;14:58–65.
76. Francis P, Bruno R, Seidman A et al. Pharmacodynamics (PD) of docetaxel (Taxotere®) in patients (PTS) with liver metastases (METS). Proc Am Soc Clin Oncol. 1994;13:138.
77. Clark PI, Slevin ML. The clinical pharmacology of etoposide and teniposide. Clin Pharmacokinet. 1997;12:223–52.
78. Slevin ML, Clark PI, Joel SP et al. A randomized trial to evaluate the effect of schedule on the activity of etoposide in small-cell lung cancer. J Clin Oncol. 1989;7:1333–40.
79. Rodman JH, Abromowitch M, Sinkul JA et al. Clinical pharmacodynamics of continuous infusion teniposide: systemic exposure as a determinant of response in a phase I trial. J Clin Oncol. 1987;5:1007–14.
80. Sinkule JA, Hutson P, Hayes FA et al. Pharmacokinetics of etoposide (VP16) in children and adolescents with refractory solid tumors. Cancer Res. 1984;44:3109–13.
81. Arbruck SG, Douglass HO, Grom WR et al. Etoposide pharmacokinetics in patients with normal and abnormal organ function. J Clin Oncol. 1986;4:1690–5.
82. D'Incalci M, Rossi C, Zucchetti M et al. Pharmacokinetics of etoposide in patients with abnormal renal and hepatic function. Cancer Res. 1986;46:2566–71.
83. Hande KR, Wolff SN, Greco FA et al. Etoposide kinetics in patients with obstructive jaundice. J Clin Oncol. 1990;8:1101–7.
84. Joel SP, Shah R, Clark PI, Slevin ML. Predicting etoposide toxicity: relationship to organ function and protein binding. J Clin Oncol. 1996;14:257–67.
85. Liu B, Earl HM, Poole C, Dunn J, Kerr DJ. Etoposide protein binding in cancer patients. Cancer Chemother Pharmacol. 1995;36:506–12.
86. Miller AA, Tolley EA, Niell HB et al. Pharmacodynamics of prolonged oral etoposide in patients with advanced non-small cell lung cancer. J Clin Oncol. 1993;11:1179–88.
87. Zucchetti M, Pagani O, Torri V et al. Clinical pharmacology of chronic oral etoposide in patients with small cell and non-small cell lung cancer. Clin Cancer Res. 1995;1:1517–24.
88. Sinkule JA, Stewart CF, Crom WR et al. Teniposide (VM26) disposition in children with leukemia. Cancer Res. 1984;44:1235–7.
89. Canal P, Bugat R, Michel C et al. Pharmacokinetics of teniposide (VM26) after IV administration in serum and malignant ascites of patients with ovarian carcinoma. Cancer Chemother Pharmacol. 1985;15:149–52.
90. Robert J, Gianni L. Pharmacokinetics and metabolism of anthracyclines. Cancer Surv. 1993;17:219–52.
91. O'Reilly SM, Richards MA, Rubens RD. Liver metastases from breast cancer: the relationship between clinical, biochemical and pathological features and survival. Eur J Cancer. 1990;26:574–77.
92. Cannizzaro R, Robieux 1, Sorio R et al. Quantitative liver function by monoethylglycinexylidide (MAGX) test in liver metastases. Gastroenterology. 1995;108:A454.
93. Sherlock S, Dooley J. Diseases of the Liver and Biliary System, 4th edn. Oxford: Blackwell, 1993;357–69.
94. Bachur NR. Adriamycin (NSC-123127) pharmacology. Cancer Chemother Rep. 1975;6:153–8.
95. Connors TA, Cox PJ, Farmer PB, Poster AB, Jarman M. Some studies of the active intermediates formed in the microsomal metabolism of cyclophosphamide and isophosphamide. Biochem Pharmacol. 1974;23:115–29.

4
Pharmacodynamics of high-dose chemotherapy

Y. NIETO

INTRODUCTION

High-dose chemotherapy (HDC) maximally capitalizes on the dose–response curves of certain antineoplastic drugs, attempting to substantially increase tumour-cell kill and improve patient outcome. The use of stem-cell support allows for dose escalation of these agents well above their myeloablative doses. While stem-cell support circumvents haematological toxicity, non-haematological organ toxicity becomes dose-limiting and can be life-threatening.

The use of pharmacokinetic (PK) measurements to direct drug dosing is common in medicine. Aminoglycosides, digoxin, and immunosuppressants are examples of drugs in which therapeutic drug monitoring (TDM) is routinely performed. In contrast, TDM is very seldom used in anticancer therapy, in spite of the inherent toxicity of chemotherapeutic agents. In the high-dose setting, where there is a potential for severe toxicity, TDM has become the holy grail of pharmacologists investigating in the field. Successful application of TDM presents several major requirements. One such requirement is identification of a therapeutically relevant target compound that can be easily measured with a short laboratory turnaround time. A second requirement is establishment of a pharmacodynamic (PD) correlation between blood levels of the target compound and a clinically meaningful endpoint, which can be related to toxicity or, less often, to tumour response or outcome. Only limited investigations of the PD effects of HDC have been reported. In this chapter I discuss current results of PD studies on HDC.

CYCLOPHOSPHAMIDE

Cyclophosphamide is widely used in HDC with autologous or allogeneic stem-cell transplantation, based on its strong immunosuppressive effect and its relative sparing of the gastrointestinal tract. At high doses its toxic profile includes cardiac necrosis, veno-occlusive disease of the liver and haemorrhagic cystitis.

Cyclophosphamide is an inactive prodrug that undergoes a complex metabolic process, summarized in Figure 1[1]. It is hydroxylated by the cytochrome P450 system to its active metabolite 4-hydroxy-cyclophosphamide, which equilibrates with its acyclic tautomer aldophosphamide. 4-Hydroxy-cyclophosphamide/ aldophosphamide enter the cell, where aldophosphamide undergoes β-elimination of acrolein to form phosphoramide mustard, the ultimate bialkylating moiety. Pharmacokinetic studies of cyclophosphamide and 4-hydroxy-cyclophosphamide/ aldophosphamide offer differing results. Slattery et al. showed an inverse association between the area under the curve (AUC) of the parent drug and its metabolites[2], whereas Chen et al. observed a direct correlation between both AUCs[3].

Inactivating reactions also play a role in cyclophosphamide metabolism. Hepatic or erythrocyte aldehyde dehydrogenase isoenzymes, particularly ALDH-1, can oxidize aldophosphamide to inactive metabolites that are excreted in the urine. In addition, cyclophosphamide can also be excreted unchanged in the urine or undergo P450-mediated side-chain oxidation to inactive compounds. Ren et al. showed a decrease in the AUC of cyclophosphamide and an increase in the AUC of 4-hydroxy-cyclophosphamide from day 1 to day 2 in patients treated with high-dose cyclophosphamide over 2 days, which appears related to an observed decrease in ALDH-1 activity during treatment[4]. It has been observed that acrolein, a degradation product of 4-hydroxy-cyclophosphamide, inhibits ALDH-1[5].

Measurement of the parent compound cyclophosphamide for TDM has important limitations. The P450-mediated hydroxylation of cyclophosphamide is subject to multiple drug–drug interactions at the microsomal level. High-dose cyclophosphamide displays nonlinear elimination kinetics, in a fashion dependent both on concentration and time[6,7]. Furthermore, a seven-fold inter-subject difference in exposure to 4-hydroxy-cyclophosphamide has been observed after cyclophosphamide–total body irradiation, where cyclophosphamide is given first, and thus is not subject to drug–radiation interactions[2].

We have analysed the PKs of cyclophosphamide in 427 patients treated at the University of Colorado with high-dose cyclophosphamide, delivered at 1875 $mg/m^2/day$ over 1 h for three consecutive days, combined with cisplatin and BCNU (STAMP-I regimen)[8]. All patients had similar pretreatment haematocrit and liver function tests, and therapy was administered under similar conditions to all of them, with the same hydration and antiemetics. We observed that neither the absolute value of cyclophosphamide AUC on day 1, nor the pattern of AUC change (increase, decrease, or minimal/no change) between days 1 and 2, predicted the pattern of change from day 2 to 3, its AUC on day 3, or its total AUC. This non-predictable intra-patient PK behaviour of cyclophosphamide calls into question the feasibility of TDM for this drug.

It has been argued that the target molecules for cyclophosphamide monitoring should not be the parent compound, but rather its active metabolites, 4-hydroxy-cyclophosphamide or aldophosphamide[9]. Study of the actual exposure to these reactive and extremely unstable intermediates has been limited in the past by analytic methodology. Real-time TDM requires rapid sample analysis with results available the next morning prior to the subsequent cyclophosphamide dose, and only recently have accurate and reproducible assays for the determination of

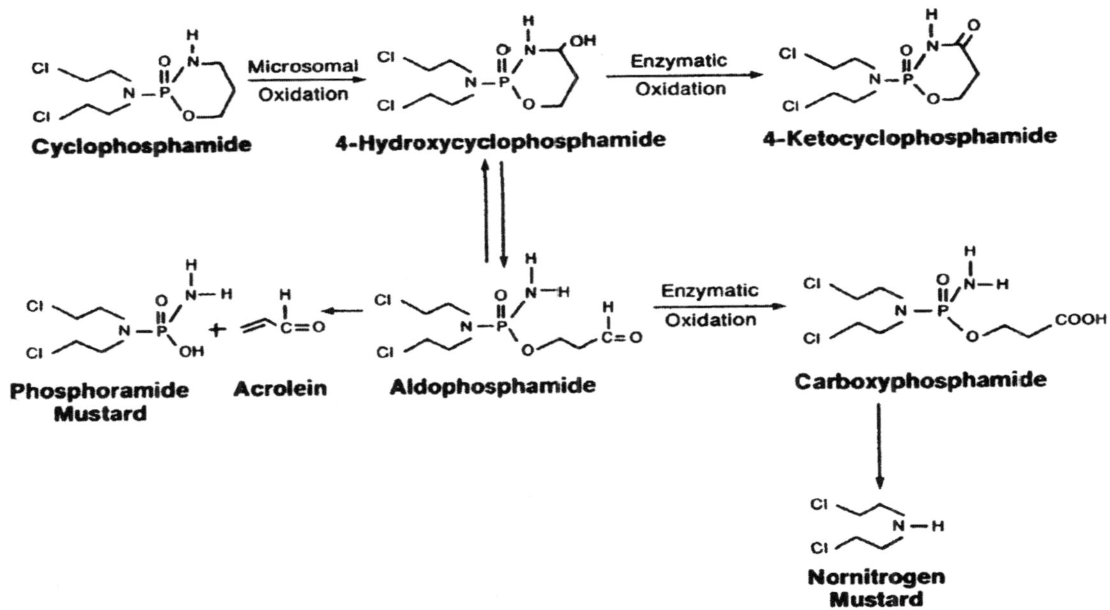

Figure 1 Metabolic pathways of cyclophosphamide

cyclophosphamide metabolites been developed. Anderson et al. described a method that includes immediate derivatization of the metabolites to form a stable oxime[10]. This assay involves gas chromatography/mass spectrometry technology and requires a specific deuterium-labelled internal standard[11]. Kalhorn et al. developed an assay to quantify 4-hydroxy-cyclophosphamide based on the bedside formation of a stable derivative[12]. The technical complexity of these assays may hamper their broad applicability. In addition, it remains unclear whether the measurement of plasma levels of 4-hydroxy-cyclophosphamide, like the quantitation of the parent drug, reflects the intracellular levels of phosphoramide mustard, the ultimate metabolite responsible for the alkylating effect.

Pharmacodynamic analyses attempting to correlate toxic and outcome endpoints with cyclophosphamide PK parameters have offered conflicting results. In a study by Ayash et al. an inverse correlation between the AUC of cyclophosphamide and both cardiotoxicity and tumour response was noted in 19 patients with metastatic breast cancer treated with high-dose cyclophosphamide, thiotepa, and carboplatin (STAMP-V regimen)[13]. Similar results were reported by Petros and colleagues in 85 patients with high-risk primary breast cancer treated with STAMP-I, including cyclophosphamide, cisplatin, and BCNU[14]. These authors observed a significant inverse relationship between the AUC of cyclophosphamide and both acute cardiac toxicity and survival.

Observations from the University of Colorado in a series of patients treated with STAMP-I showed no correlation between the total AUC of cyclophosphamide and the occurrence of toxic death, cardiotoxicity, post-transplant relapse, or survival in any of the groups analysed: stage II/III breast cancer (n = 115), metastatic breast cancer (n = 163), and non-Hodgkin's lymphoma (NHL) (n = 50)[8,15,16]. In the subgroup of patients with breast cancer and minimal metastatic disease the AUC of cisplatin (Figure 2A), but not of BCNU (Figure 2B) or cyclophosphamide (Figure 2C), directly correlated with incidence of treatment-related death[15].

There is an ongoing controversy on whether cyclophosphamide is an adequate drug for high-dose therapy. While cyclophosphamide has been a mainstay of HDC, there is increasing scepticism regarding its value for dose escalation with stem-cell support. Two large randomized trials conducted by the National Surgical Adjuvant Breast and Bowel Project (NSABP) tested the escalation of both dose intensity and total cumulative dose of cyclophosphamide, combined with adriamycin, in the adjuvant treatment of more than 4800 node-positive breast cancer patients[17,18]. No improvements in DFS or OS were observed after substantial increases of up to four-fold in the dose intensity (2400 mg/m^2 every 3 weeks) or total dose (9600 mg/m^2 over four cycles) of this drug.

These results contrast sharply with the steep dose–response effect clearly present with cyclophosphamide metabolites *in vitro*. A possible explanation for this discrepancy stems from the complexity of the pharmacology and metabolic pathways of cyclophosphamide. Busse et al.[19] treated 12 patients with four courses of cyclophosphamide at 500 mg/m^2, followed by one course of high-dose cyclophosphamide at 100 mg/kg. An increase in the renal excretion of the inactive metabolites carboxyphosphamide and dechloroethylcyclophosphamide was observed, with a decrease in the metabolic clearance of the parent

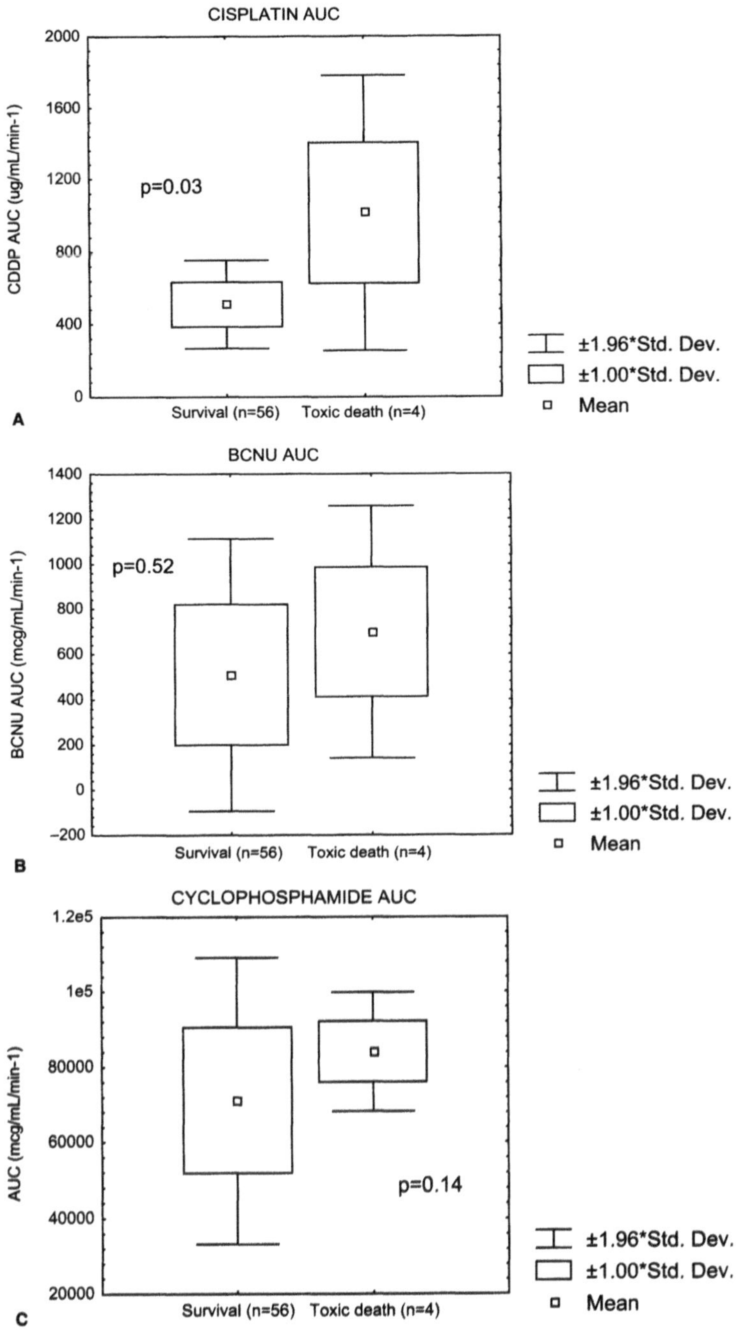

Figure 2 Pharmacodynamic analysis of cisplatin (**A**), BCNU (**B**), and cyclophosphamide (**C**) in the phase II study of HDC in patients with metastatic breast cancer and no evidence of disease (NED), conducted at the University of Colorado BMT Program

compound towards its active metabolites. This intrapatient shift from activating toward inactivating reactions indicates saturation of bioactivating enzymes at the higher doses.

Dockham et al. showed a three-fold inter-individual variation in the erythrocyte fraction of ALDH-1, an enzyme that seems to play an important role in the detoxification of 4-hydroxy-cyclophosphamide[20]. Thus, variations in the haematocrit may also change drug disposition and exposure of tumour cells to the active metabolites.

While cyclophosphamide is still considered by some authors as a time-honoured and worthy drug for high-dose therapy, the results of the NSABP randomized trials raise serious concerns about its inclusion in high-dose regimens, particularly for breast cancer.

MELPHALAN

Based on its toxic profile and steep dose–response curve, melphalan has long been included in HDC combinations with stem-cell support. Myeloma probably constitutes the most successful application of melphalan-based HDC. High-dose melphalan, either as single agent at 200 mg/m^2, or at a lower dose (140 mg/m^2) combined with total-body irradiation (TBI), constitutes the standard of care for patients with responding myeloma[21].

Further dose escalation of melphalan has been explored as a means to increase its cytotoxicity. Administration of melphalan at 220 mg/m^2 has been shown to be tolerable and active in myeloma patients who had relapsed after prior HDC[22]. Phillips and colleagues have reported the interim results of an ongoing phase I study of melphalan combined with amifostine, a glutathione analogue with selectivity for normal cells[23]. No dose-limiting toxicities have been encountered at a dose of melphalan of 300 mg/m^2.

Over the past decade a number of phase II and III studies have evaluated melphalan-containing HDC regimens, combining this drug with cyclophosphamide and mitoxantrone for breast cancer, or etoposide, cytarabine and BCNU for lymphomas. Development of HDC combinations of melphalan with novel drugs is in progress.

While there has been considerable concern regarding the use of high-dose melphalan, given its potential for long-term carcinogenesis, recent data suggest that the preceding standard-dose therapy is more likely the cause of secondary leukaemia or myelodysplastic syndrome after melphalan-containing HDCT[24,25]. In addition, in a retrospective analysis of 725 patients with haematological malignancies treated at a single institution and followed over 26 years, the use of melphalan/TBI did not appear to be associated with a higher risk of second malignant neoplasms than cyclophosphamide/TBI[26].

The dose-limiting toxicity of high-dose melphalan is gastrointestinal[27]. There is a large intra- and inter-patient variability in absorption of the oral form, both at standard and high doses[28,29]. Alberts et al. studied the PKs of intravenous administration, which avoids the problem of inconsistent oral absorption[30]. Melphalan does not require metabolic activation. About 15% of the drug is excreted intact in the urine. Inactive monohydroxy and dihydroxy metabolites appear in plasma within minutes of the drug administration. In a study using intravenous melphalan the incidence of severe myelosuppression increased in patients with BUN levels above 30 mg/dl, suggesting that these patients may have altered drug excretion[31]. Melphalan PKs remain linear when delivered at high doses. After high-dose therapy the mean peak cerebrospinal fluid concentrations may reach 10% of the corresponding plasma levels[32], and the drug may achieve levels in cerebrospinal fluid which are associated with effective *in-vitro* cell killing[33,34]. A PK study in patients receiving high-dose melphalan showed AUCs that ranged from 4.85 to 19.86 mg/h/L in patients with creatinine clearance above 40 mg/dl[35]. The use of high-dose melphalan appears to be safe in patients with renal failure[36].

Tranchand et al. showed in a small group of seven patients that the AUC of low-dose melphalan could be accurately predicted by a test dose[37]. In a follow-up study this group showed that PK-directed dosing was possible[38]. Current research is exploring TDM of high-dose melphalan, using either the test-dose approach in single-administration schedules, or dose modifications based on the PKs of the first dose, when the drug is delivered in multiple administrations.

THIOTEPA

Thiotepa is another alkylating agent that has been used in anticancer therapy for many years. Its current systemic use is largely limited to HDC combinations for breast or ovarian cancer. Thiotepa is included in the experimental arm of several large randomized phase III trials comparing high-dose to standard-dose combinations for breast cancer at various stages, which either have been completed[39], or are still under way[40,41].

These thiotepa-containing HDC regimens also include cyclophosphamide, with or without carboplatin (as in STAMP-V), cisplatin, or BCNU. The potential of cyclophosphamide to interact with other drugs at the P450 cytochromes was discussed previously. Recently, it was observed that when cyclophosphamide and thiotepa are given concurrently, as in STAMP-V, thiotepa exposure is significantly decreased[42].

BUSULFAN

The use of busulfan, a bifunctional alkylator, is primarily restricted to HDC with autologous or allogeneic bone marrow transplantation for haematological malignancies, particularly of the myeloid lineage. This approach exploits its marked cytotoxicity against myeloid cells and its marked dose–response effect.

Until recently busulfan was available only in an oral formulation. Oral busulfan has an irregular bioavailability and variable PKs. Given its large potential for severe toxicity, particularly to the liver, its erratic absorption is of concern. Grochow and colleagues showed a direct correlation between its total AUC and the incidence of severe hepatic toxicity[43]. These authors showed that prospective TDM of oral busulfan after the first dose reduces the incidence of veno-occlusive disease of the liver. This has arguably become one of the most successful applications of the principles of TDM to clinical practice in HDC. In a pharmacodynamic analysis by Slattery and colleagues a low steady-state concentration of busulfan was associated with a higher incidence of post-transplant relapse in patients with chronic myelogenous leukaemia[44].

An intravenous preparation of busulfan was recently formulated[45]. Regimens containing high-dose intravenous busulfan have subsequently been tested in clinical trials for myeloid malignancies[46] and NHL[47]. Intravenous busulfan appears to provide reliable systemic drug exposure, decreased inter-individual and inter-dose PK variability, and reduced toxicity, when compared to the oral formulation[48]. Recent data suggest the reliability of PK-directed dosing of intravenous busulfan used at high doses[49].

BCNU (CARMUSTINE)

BCNU is currently used at standard doses (100–200 mg/m^2) in the treatment of brain tumours and melanoma. BCNU-related myelosuppression, characteristically delayed and with marked selectivity for early precursors, is its major toxicity at conventional doses. This effect appears to be related to the low content of the detoxifying enzyme O^6-alkylguanine-DNA alkyltransferase in early haematopoietic precursors[50].

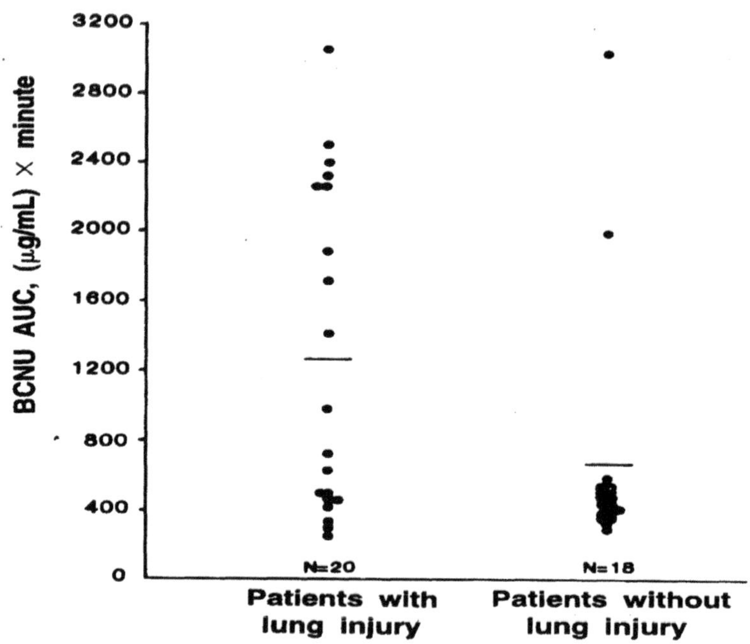

Figure 3 Scatter plot showing BCNU AUC values of patients who experienced toxic lung injury compared with those who did not experience it ($p < 0.05$)

A steep dose–response effect and favourable toxic profile at conventional doses provided the rationale for inclusion of BCNU in HDC regimens, combined with cyclophosphamide and cisplatin for breast cancer (STAMP-I), or etoposide, ara-C, and melphalan (BEAM), for lymphoma.

In the early phase I trials of single-agent BCNU with stem-cell support, liver toxicity and encephalopathy were dose-limiting. In contrast, its most prominent side-effect when part of the STAMP-I regimen is steroid-responsive interstitial pneumonitis, which occurs in more than 50% of patients. Jones and colleagues analysed patients treated at the University of Colorado BMT Program, and observed a direct correlation between the AUC of BCNU and the risk of developing pulmonary toxicity (Figure 3)[51]. These authors also showed that pretreatment with cisplatin and cyclophosphamide produces large increases in both the value and the variability of the AUC of BCNU[52].

PACLITAXEL

The dose-limiting toxicity of paclitaxel infused over 24 h is myelosuppression[53]. A phase I dose-escalation study of paclitaxel over 24 h combined with high doses of cyclophosphamide and cisplatin, with autologous stem-cell support, was conducted at the University of Colorado BMT Program[54]. A dose of 775 mg/m^2 of paclitaxel was identified as its MTD, which represents a three-fold increment over its unsupported MTD in this schedule of administration. A significant, albeit weak, correlation was found between the severity of peripheral neuropathy and the AUC ($r = 0.54$, $p = 0.00001$) and peak serum levels ($r = 0.57$, $p < 0.00005$) of paclitaxel. An association was also found between the severity of mucositis and the AUC ($r = 0.48$, $p < 0.001$) and peak concentrations ($r = 0.46$, $p < 0.001$) of paclitaxel.

A significant toxicity observed with high-dose paclitaxel is acute encephalopathy. Occurrence of this side-effect did not correlate with any PK parameter in an analysis of 129 patients treated with paclitaxel-containing HDC at the University of Colorado[55].

DOCETAXEL

Docetaxel is a potent drug against a variety of solid tumours, most notably breast cancer. Preclinical data suggest a dose-dependent and schedule-independent antitumour activity. Neutropenia is its dose-limiting toxicity at its standard MTD of 100 mg/m^2. A phase I trial conducted at the University of Colorado explored the dose escalation of docetaxel with stem-cell support, above its myeloablative dose, in combination with high doses of melphalan and carboplatin[56]. The MTD of docetaxel was reached at 450 mg/m^2, infused over 2 h. Pharmacokinetic studies showed linear increases of AUC ($r = 0.74$, $p < 0.00005$) (Figure 4A) and C_{max} ($r = 0.82$, $p<0.000005$) (Figure 4B) with dose, but not of its β-half life ($r = -0.37$, $p = 0.09$) (Figure 3C). The observed PK linearity of high-dose docetaxel is remarkable considering that the drug undergoes enzymatic metabolism in the liver, and reflects non-saturation of its metabolic pathways.

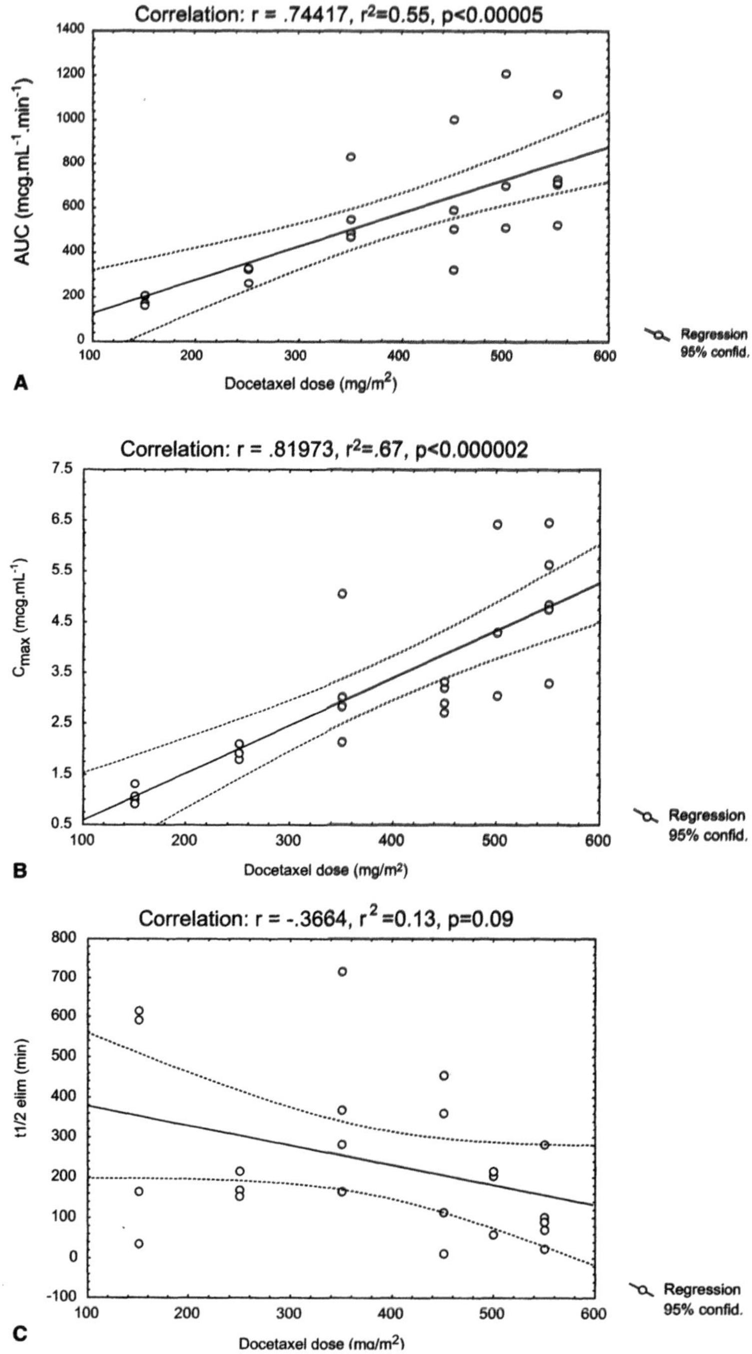

Figure 4 Linearity of high-dose docetaxel pharmacokinetics: correlation between dose and AUC (**A**), dose and C_{max} (**B**), and dose and elimination half-life (**C**)

Pharmacodynamic analyses showed correlations between the observed severity of polyneuropathy and the measured AUC ($r = 0.86$, $p = 0.000001$) (Figure 4), or C_{max} ($r = 0.82$, $p < 0.000001$) (Figure 5). Likewise, the associations between the severity of stomatitis and AUC ($r = 0.62$, $p = 0.01$) (Figure 6) or C_{max} ($r = 0.6$, $p = 0.001$) (Figure 7) were statistically significant. In both cases the PD correlations were stronger evaluating the measured PK parameters than using the administered dose of docetaxel.

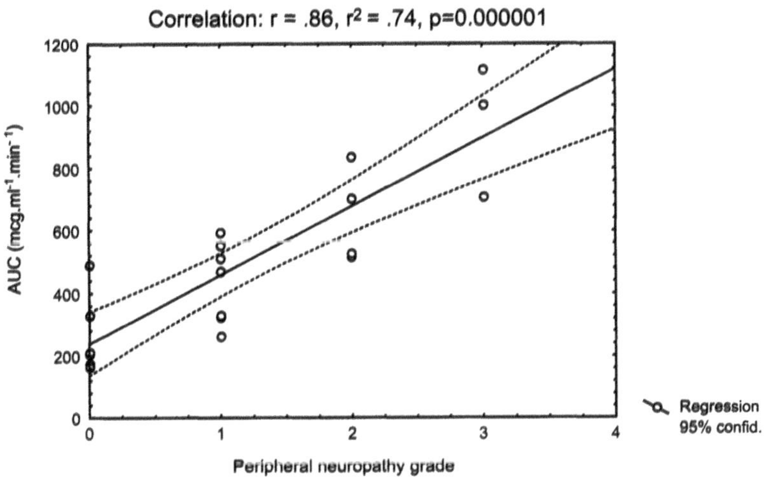

Figure 5 Correlation between the severity of peripheral neuropathy observed in a phase I trial of docetaxel conducted at the University of Colorado BMT Program and the measured AUC of this compound

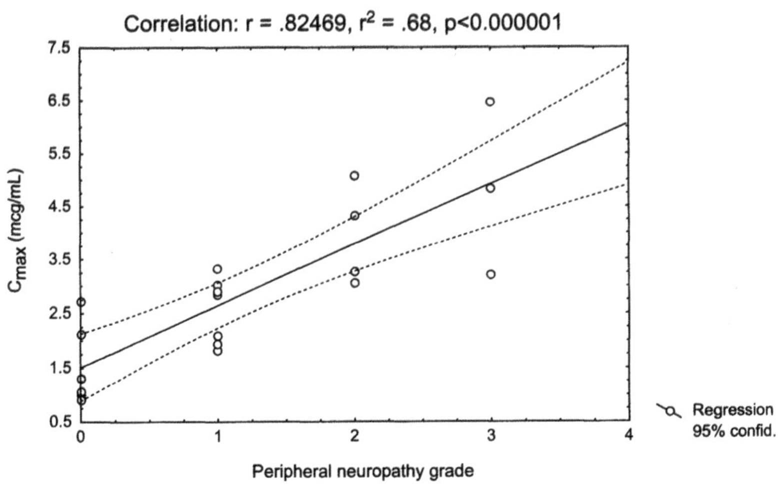

Figure 6 Correlation between the severity of peripheral neuropathy and the C_{max} of docetaxel

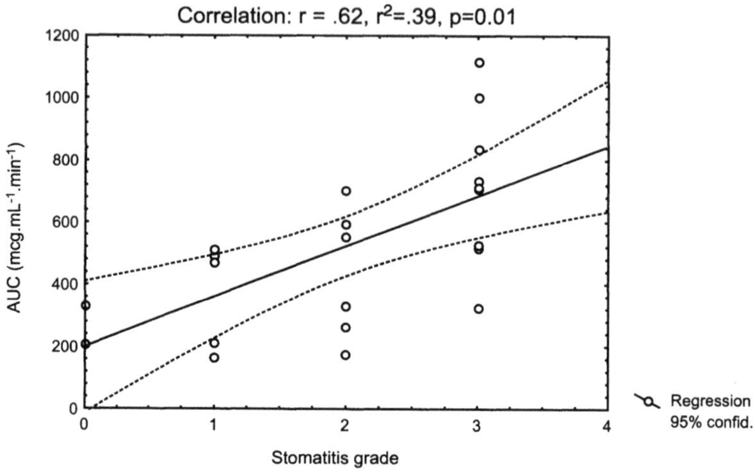

Figure 7 Correlation between the severity of mucositis and the AUC of docetaxel

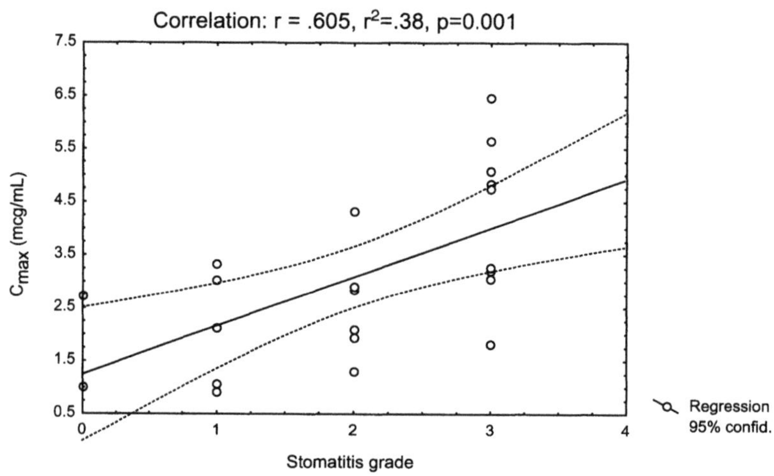

Figure 8 Correlation between mucositis severity and the C_{max} of docetaxel

CONCLUSIONS

Phamacodynamic studies performed to date have shown that PK parameters of some of the drugs that compose the high-dose armamentarium correlate with clinical endpoints. Pharmacodynamic observations such as these are a previous requirement to successful application of prospective TDM. The goal of this strategy is reduction in the variability of drug exposure by the application of PK-directed dosing, which may decrease the variability in toxic or therapeutic outcomes. Studies are in progress that pursue TDM of drugs employed in HDC, such as busulfan or melphalan.

References

1. Colvin OM. An overview of cyclophosphamide development and clinical applications. Curr Pharmaceut Design. 1999;5:555–60.
2. Slattery JT, Kalhorn TF, McDonald GB et al. Conditioning regimen-dependent disposition of cyclophosphamide and hydroxycyclophosphamide in human marrow transplantation patients. J Clin Oncol. 1996;14:1484–94.
3. Chen T-L, Kennedy MJ, Anderson LW et al. Nonlinear pharmacokinetics of cyclophosphamide and 4-hydroxycyclophosphamide/aldophosphamide in patients with metastatic breast cancer receiving high-dose chemotherapy followed by autologous bone marrow transplantation. Drug Metab Dispos. 1997;25:544–51.
4. Ren S, Kalhorn TF, McDonald GB, Anasetti C, Appelbaum FR, Slattery JT. Pharmacokinetics of cyclophosphamide and its metabolites in bone marrow transplantation patients. Cancer Chemother Pharmacol. 1998;64:289–301.
5. Ren S, Kalhorn TF, Slattery JT. Inhibition of human aldehyde dehydrogenase 1 by the 4-hydroxycyclophosphamide degradation product acrolein. Drug Metab Dispos. 1999;27:133–7.
6. Grochow LB, Colvin OM. Clinical pharmacokinetics of cyclophosphamide. Clin Pharmacokinet. 1980;4:380–94.
7. Chen T-L, Passos-Coelho JL, Noe DA et al. Nonlinear pharmacokinetics of cyclophosphamide in patients with metastatic breast cancer receiving high-dose chemotherapy followed by autologous bone marrow transplantation. Cancer Res. 1995;550:810–16.
8. Nieto Y, Xu X, Cagnoni PJ et al. Nonpredictable pharmacokinetic behavior of high-dose cyclophosphamide in combination with cisplatin and 1,3-bis(2-chloroethyl)-nitrosourea. Clin Cancer Res. 1999;5:747–51.
9. Petros WP, Colvin OM. Metabolic jeopardy with high-dose cyclophosphamide? – Not so fast. Clin Cancer Res. 1999;5:723–4.
10. Anderson LW, Ludeman SM, Colvin OM, Grochow LB, Strong JM. Quantitation of 4-hydroxycyclophosphamide/aldophosphamide in whole blood. J Chromatogr B. 1995;667:247–57.
11. Ludeman SM, Shulamn-Roskes EM, Wong KK et al. Oxime derivatives of the intermediary oncostatic metabolites of cyclophosphamide and ifosfamide: synthesis and deuterium labeling for applications to metabolite quantification. J Pharm Sci. 1995;84:393–8.
12. Kalhorn TF, Ren S, Howald WN, Lawrence RF, Slattery JT. Analysis of cyclophosphamide and five metabolites from human plasma using liquid chromatography–mass spectrometry and gas chromatography–nitrogen–phosphorus detection. J Chromatogr B Biomed Sci Appl. 1999;732:287–98.
13. Ayash LJ, Wright JE, Tretyakov O et al. Cyclophosphamide pharmacokinetics: correlation with cardiac toxicity and tumor response. J Clin Oncol. 1992;10:995–1000.
14. Petros WP, Broadwater G, Berry D et al. Correlation of high-dose cyclophosphamide (CPA), cisplatin (CDDP), and carmustine (BCNU) pharmacokinetics (PK) to response and toxicity in patients with primary breast cancer. Proc Am Soc Clin Oncol. 1997;16:216a.
15. Nieto Y, Cagnoni PJ, Shpall EJ et al. Phase II trial of high-dose chemotherapy with autologous stem cell transplant for stage IV breast cancer with minimal metastatic disease. Clin Cancer Res. 1999;5:1731–7.
16. Nieto Y, Cagnoni PJ, Bearman SI et al. Cardiac toxicity following high-dose cyclophosphamide, cisplatin, and BCNU (STAMP-I) in breast cancer patients. Biol Blood Marrow Transplant. 2000;6:198–203.
17. Fisher B, Anderson S, Wickerham DL et al. Increased intensification and total dose of cyclophosphamide in a doxorubicin–cyclophosphamide regimen for the treatment of primary breast cancer: findings from National Surgical Adjuvant Breast and Bowel Project B-22. J Clin Oncol. 1997;15:1858–69.
18. Fisher B, Anderson S, DeCillis A et al. Further evaluation of intensified and increased total dose of cyclophosphamide for the treatment of primary breast cancer: findings from National Surgical Adjuvant Breast and Bowel Project B-25. J Clin Oncol. 1999;17:3374–88.
19. Busse D, Busch FW, Bohnenstengel F et al. Dose escalation of cyclophosphamide in patients with breast cancer: consequences for pharmacokinetics and metabolism. J Clin Oncol. 1997;15:1885–96.
20. Dockham PA, Sreerama L, Sladek NE. Relative contribution of human erythrocyte aldehyde dehydrogenase to the systemic detoxification of the oxazaphosphorines. Drug Metab Dispos. 1997;25:1436–41.

21. Attal M, Harousseau JL, Stoppa AM et al. A prospective, randomized trial of autologous bone marrow transplantation and chemotherapy in multiple myeloma. Intergroupe Francais du Myelome. N Engl J Med. 1996;335:91–7.
22. Moreau P, Milpied N, Mahe B et al. Melphalan 220 mg/m^2 followed by peripheral blood stem cell transplantation in 27 patients with advanced multiple myeloma. Bone Marrow Transplant. 1999;23:1003–6.
23. Phillips GL, Hale GA, Howard DS et al. Amifostine cytoprotection of escalating doses of melphalan and autologous hematopoietic stem cell transplantation: a phase I–II study. Proc Am Soc Clin Oncol. 2000;19:49a.
24. Govindarajan R, Jagannath S, Flick JT et al. Preceding standard therapy is the likely cause of MDS after autotransplants for multiple myeloma. Br J Haematol. 1996;95:349–53.
25. Pedersen-Bjergaard J, Pedersen M, Myhre J, Geisler C. High risk of therapy-related leukemia after BEAM chemotherapy and autologous stem cell transplantation for previously treated lymphomas is mainly related to primary chemotherapy and not to the BEAM-transplantation procedure. Leukemia. 1997;11:1654–60.
26. Kulkarni S, Powles R, Treleaven J et al. Melphalan/TBI is not more carcinogenic than cyclophosphamide/TBI for transplant conditioning: follow-up of 725 patients from a single centre over a period of 26 years. Bone Marrow Transplant. 2000;25:365–70.
27. Lazarus HM, Herzig RH, Graham-Pole J et al. Intensive melphalan chemotherapy and cryopreserved autologous bone marrow transplantation for the treatment of refractory cancer. J Clin Oncol. 1983;1:359–67.
28. Alberts DS, Chang SY, Cheng HSG et al. Oral melphalan kinetics. Clin Pharmacol Ther. 1979;26:737–45.
29. Choi KE, Ratain MJ, Williams SF et al. Plasma pharmacokinetics of high-dose oral melphalan in patients treated with trialkylator chemotherapy and autologous bone marrow reinfusion. Cancer Res. 1989;49:1318–21.
30. Alberts DS, Chang SY, Chen HSG et al. Kinetics of intravenous melphalan. Clin Pharmacol Ther. 1979;26:73–80.
31. Cornwell GO, Pajak TF, McIntyre OR et al. Influence of renal failure on myelosuppressive effects of melphalan: Cancer and Leukemia Group B experience. Cancer Treat Rep. 1982;66:475–81.
32. Lazarus HM, Herzig RH, Graham-Pole J et al. Intensive melphalan chemotherapy and cryopreserved autologous bone marrow transplantation for the treatment of refractory cancer. J Clin Oncol. 1983;1:359–67.
33. Goodman GE, Chang SY, Alberts DS. The antitumor activity of melphalan and its hydrolysis products. Proc Am Assoc Cancer Res. 1980;21:301.
34. Salmon SE, Hamburger AW, Soehnlen B et al. Quantitation of differential sensitivity of human-tumor stem cells to anticancer drugs. N Engl J Med. 1978;298:1321–7.
35. Tricot G, Alberts DS, Johnson C et al. Safety of autotransplants with high-dose melphalan in renal failure: a pharmacokinetic and toxicity study. Clin Cancer Res. 1996;2:947–52.
36. Tricot G, Alberts DS, Johnson C et al. Safety of autotransplants with high-dose melphalan in renal failure: a pharmacokinetic and toxicity study. Clin Cancer Res. 1996;2:947–52.
37. Tranchand B, Ploin Y-D, Minuit M-P et al. High-dose melphalan dosage adjustment: possibility of using a test dose. Cancer Chemother Pharmacol. 1989;23:95–100.
38. Ploin DY, Tranchand B, Guastalla J-P et al. Pharmacokinetically guided dosing for intravenous melphalan: a pilot study in patients with advanced ovarian adenocarcinoma. Eur J Cancer. 1992;28A:1311–15.
39. Stadtmauer EA, O'Neill A, Goldstein LJ et al. Conventional-dose chemotherapy compared with high-dose chemotherapy plus autologous hematopoietic stem-cell transplantation for metastatic breast cancer. N Engl J Med. 2000;342:1069–76.
40. Rodenhuis S, Bontenbal M, Beex L et al. Randomized phase III trial of high-dose chemotherapy with cyclophosphamide, thiotepa and carboplatin in operable breast cancer with 4 or more axillary lymph nodes. Proc Am Soc Clin Oncol. 2000;19:74a.
41. Scandinavian Study Group 9401. Results from a randomized adjuvant breast cancer study with high dose chemotherapy with CTCb supported by autologous bone marrow stem cells versus dose escalated and tailored FEC therapy. Proc Am Soc Clin Oncol. 1999;18:2a.
42. Huitema AD, Tibben MM, Kerbusch T, Zwikker JW, Rodenhuis S, Beijnen JH. Simultaneous determination of N,N′,N″-triethylenthiophosphoramide, cyclophosphamide and some of their

metabolites in plasma using capillary gas chromatography. J Chromatogr B Biomed Sci Appl. 1998;16:177–86.
43. Grochow LB, Piantadosi S, Santos G, Jones R. Busulfan dose adjustment decreases the risk of venoocclusive disease in patients undergoing bone marrow transplantation. Proc Am Assoc Cancer Res. 1992;33:200.
44. Slattery JT, Clift RA, Buckner CD et al. Marrow transplantation for chronic myeloid leukemia: the influence of plasma busulfan levels on the outcome of transplantation. Blood. 1997;89:3055–60.
45. Bhagwatwar HP, Phadungpojna S, Chow DS, Andersson BS. Formulation and stability of busulfan for intravenous administration in high-dose chemotherapy. Cancer Chemother Pharmacol. 1996;37:401–8.
46. Andersson BS, Gajewski J, Donato M et al. Allogeneic stem cell transplantation (BMT) for AML and MDS following i.v. busulfan and cyclophosphamide (i.v. BuCy). Bone Marrow Transplant. 2000;26(Suppl. 2):S35–8.
47. Andersson BS, Tran H, Mirza N et al. Stem cell transplantation for non-Hodgkin's lymphomas after IV busulfan and cyclophosphamide. Proc Am Soc Clin Oncol. 1999;18:47a.
48. Andersson BS, Madden T, Tran HT et al. Acute safety and pharmacokinetics of intravenous busulfan when used with oral busulfan and cyclophosphamide as pretransplantation conditioning therapy: a phase I therapy. Biol Blood Marrow Transplant. 2000;6:548–54.
49. Perry SL, Salzman DE, Carabasi MH, Vaughan WP. Pharmacokinetically based individualized IV busulfan therapy in marrow transplant regimens. Biol Blood Marrow Transplant. 2000;6:155a.
50. Gerson SL, Phillips W, Kastan M et al. Human CD34 hematopoietic progenitors have low, cytokine-unresponsive O6-alkylguanine-DNA alkyltransferase and are sensitive to O6-benzylguanine plus BCNU. Blood. 1996;88:1649.
51. Jones RB, Matthes SM, Shpall EJ et al. Acute lung injury following treatment with high-dose cyclophosphamide, cisplatin, and carmustine: pharmacodynamic evaluation of carmustine. J Natl Cancer Inst. 1993;85:640–7.
52. Jones RB, Matthes S, Kemme D et al. Cyclophosphamide, cisplatin and carmustine: pharmacokinetics of carmustine following multiple alkylating-agent interactions. Cancer Chemother Pharmacol. 1994;35:59–63.
53. Rowinsky EK, Eisenhauer EA, Chaudhry V et al. Clinical toxicities encountered with paclitaxel (Taxol). Semin Oncol. 1993;20:1–15.
54. Stemmer SM, Cagnoni PJ, Shpall EJ et al. High-dose paclitaxel, cyclophosphamide, and cisplatin with autologous hematopoietic progenitor-cell support: a phase I trial. J Clin Oncol. 1996;14:1463–72.
55. Nieto Y, Cagnoni PJ, Bearman SI et al. Acute encephalopathy: a new toxicity associated with high-dose paclitaxel. Clin Cancer Res. 1999;5:501–6.
56. Nieto Y, Cagnoni PJ, Shpall EJ et al. Phase I trial of docetaxel combined with fixed doses of melphalan and carboplatin, with peripheral blood progenitor cell support in refractory malignancies. Proc Am Soc Clin Oncol. 2000;19:56a.

Section II
Chemotherapeutic agents in the individual patient

5
Interactions of cytostatic drugs

W. KÄMMERER

INTRODUCTION

According to the latest research, interactions between drugs are responsible for one-third of all adverse drug effects and cause about half of the related costs in Germany. Recent examples (cerivastatin, cisapride, mibefradil) clearly show the clinical relevance of drug interactions. However, even herbal substances and nutritional components can interact with drugs.

Due to their small therapeutic range and high toxicity, cytostatic drugs are predisposed to interactions. A decrease in efficacy and an insufficient antitumoral effect present a considerable risk to the patient, while similar risks accompany an increase in efficacy and considerable toxicity.

This chapter primarily deals with pharmacokinetic interactions between cytostatic drugs and other medications. They can occur by:

1. influencing resorption,
2. influencing bonding to plasma proteins or tissue,
3. influencing elimination by modifying biotransformation or modifying excretion.

The most important interactions occur in the area of elimination. This involves cytochrome P450 monooxygenases (CYP) and transport proteins (among others p-glycoprotein).

CYTOCHROME P450 MONOOXYGENASES (CYP)

This is a family of haemoproteins which plays an important role in the metabolism of numerous and structurally differentiated lipophilic foreign substances. Based on the homology of their amino acid sequences the individual isoforms are subdivided into families and subfamilies. However, they each have characteristic spectra of catalytic activity and substrate specificity, parts of which overlap. There are three CYP gene families (CYP1, CYP2, CYP3) which are particularly responsible for the hepatic metabolism of drugs.

CYP3A (CYP3A4 and CYP3A5) and CYP2C (CYP2C8, CYP2C9, CYP2C18 and CYP2C19) are the most common subfamilies, which make up approximately 50% and 20% respectively, of the total activity of CYP in the human liver. Yet CYP3A4 is the most common single CYP isoenzyme (about 50% of total activity). CYP isoenzymes are present not only in the liver but also in other organs. The expression of CYP in the intestinal wall is particularly important in drug pharmacokinetics. This may lead to the metabolic inactivation of previously absorbed medicinal agents during their passage through the intestinal wall to the portal venous blood stream.

Thus, intestinal CYP enzymes play an important role in the first-pass metabolism of drugs and may considerably reduce their oral bioavailability.

Known inhibitors of CYP enzymes are: amiodarone, azole antimycotic agents, cimetidine, calcium antagonists (among others diltiazem, nifedipine, verapamil), grapefruit juice, macrolide antibiotics, SSRI (fluoxetine, fluvoxamine) and anti-HIV medications, isoniazid. Known inducers of CYP are: barbiturates, carbamazepine and oxcarbazepine dexamethasones, St John's Wort, phenytoin, rifampin/rifabutin.

TRANSPORT PROTEINS

Another mechanism which is important for the bioavailability and intracellular elimination of drugs is affinity to transport proteins. The family of ABC transport proteins is a heterogeneous group of membrane-based proteins whose function is the transmembranous transport of numerous xenobiotics. Probably the best known representative of this group is p-glycoprotein; if its expression in carcinoma cells is up-regulated, cytostatic drugs may increasingly be released from these cells, which leads to the phenomenon of 'multi-drug resistance' in carcinomas.

In the gastrointestinal tract p-glycoprotein inhibits absorption by pumping drugs back into the intestinal lumen. In the liver p-glycoprotein causes increased elimination into the gallbladder; in the kidneys renal elimination is promoted. In addition, p-glycoprotein influences the blood–brain barrier, where it counteracts the intracerebral penetration of substances.

P-glycoprotein exhibits a very broad substrate specificity; many drugs are substrates for CYP isoenzymes as well as for p-glycoprotein.

P-glycoprotein can be induced or inhibited. An inhibition of p-glycoprotein leads to a higher intracellular drug concentration, which may be of therapeutic use in the future.

Known inhibitors are: amiodarone, chinidine, cyclosporine, clarithromycin, erythromycin, grapefruit juice, itraconazole, ketoconazole, ritonavir, saquinavir, SSRI (fluoxetine, paroxetine), verapamil. Known inducers are St John's wort and rifampin.

Interactions may be expected when cytostatic drugs are substrates of these enzymes, and when these cytostatic drugs are used in combination with drugs which may inhibit or induce these enzyme systems.

The following cytostatic drugs are substrates, inducers or inhibitors of CYP: capecitabine, cyclophosphamide, dacarbazine, docetaxel, etoposide, ifosfamide, imatinib, irinotecan, paclitaxel, vinca alkaloids.

The following cytostatic drugs are known substrates of p-glycoprotein: daunorubicin, docetaxel, doxorubicin, etoposide, mitoxantrone, paclitaxel, teniposide, vinca alkaloids.

KNOWN, CLINICALLY RELEVANT INTERACTIONS OF CYTOSTATIC DRUGS

Cyclophosphamide, ifosfamide

These are activated through CYP. Caution is advised when administering these at the same time as CYP inducers such as phenobarbital or phenytoin, since an increase in toxicity may occur. The clinical relevance of these potential interactions remains unclear. Conversely, enzyme inhibitors are theoretically able to reduce the efficacy of cyclophosphamide.

When given simultaneously with ondansetron, cyclophosphamide clearance is increased by 17%. When given simultaneously with allopurinol its levels in plasma increase and the duration of cyclophosphamide efficacy is prolonged, resulting in increased toxicity. Simultaneous application should therefore be avoided.

Docetaxel

Docetaxel is metabolized by CYP3A4 and is a substrate of p-glycoprotein. No clinical studies of interactions are available. However, caution is advised when administering CYP and p glycoprotein inhibitors or inducers at the same time.

The elimination of docetaxel *in vitro* is considerably inhibited by cyclosporine, erythromycin and ketoconazole.

Doxorubicin

Doxorubicin is metabolized by CYP and is a substrate of p-glycoprotein. Barbiturates reduce efficacy via CYP induction.

Digoxin levels are probably lowered due to an influence on p-glycoprotein. Severe neurotoxic side-effects were reported when doxorubicin was given at the same time as cyclosporine. The reason for this is probably the inhibition of p-glycoprotein by cyclosporine.

Case reports apparently suggest that plasma levels of doxorubicin and its active metabolite doxorubicinol are increased after combined use with paclitaxel. The probable reason for this is the inhibition of CYP enzymes or p-glycoprotein by paclitaxel.

Epirubicin

In prolonged use, cimetidine increases the AUC of epirubicin by 50% via CYP inhibition; thus it should not be used at the same time as epirubicin.

Etoposide

Etoposide is metabolized by CYP3A4 and is a substrate of p-glycoprotein. If used simultaneously with a high dosage of cyclosporine a considerable increase in serum levels of etoposide is seen as a result of the inhibition of p-glycoprotein-aided elimination.

In general, caution is advised when CYP and p-glycoprotein inhibitors or inducers are used at the same time.

Fluorouracil and its pro-drugs

5-FU, tegafur

Metronidazole inhibits the clearance of 5-FU. An AUC increase of 35% together with a corresponding increase in toxicity are reported.

Capecitabine

This is metabolized by CYP. If administered simultaneously with oral anticoagulants, haemorrhage may occur due to CYP2C9 inhibition by capecitabine. When phenytoin is administered simultaneously, the inhibition of CYP2C9 causes an increased phenytoin toxicity.

Imatinib

This is a substrate of, and even inhibits, the CYP enzymes 3A4, 2D6, 2C9 and 2C19. If administered together with CYP inhibitors such as ketoconazole, itraconazole, erythromycin, and clarithromycin, a considerable increase in the imatinib concentration occurs (increase in the mean C_{max} and AUC of imatinib by 26% and 40% respectively). If given simultaneously with CYP inducers such as phenytoin (documented), carbamazepine, rifampin, phenobarbital, and St John's wort, the serum concentration decreases, resulting in a loss of efficacy.

Caution is also advised when administering this drug simultaneously with CYP substrates such as statines, oral anticoagulants or paracetamol.

Thus, when administered simultaneously with simvastatin (CYP3A4), for example, an increase in the AUC and C_{max} by a factor of 2 and 3.5 respectively may occur. If the drug is administered at the same time as warfarin a PT check is required. Paracetamol should not be used due to the inhibition of CYP2D6 by imatinib.

Irinotecan

Irinotecan is metabolized through CYP3A4 and is a substrate of p-glycoprotein. Clinically relevant interactions with the CYP and p-glycoprotein inhibitor ketoconazole (efficacy is increased) as well as with the CYP and p-glycoprotein inducer St John's wort (loss of efficacy) are known to exist.

6-Mercaptopurine, azathioprine

If 6-MP or azathioprine is administered at the same time as allopurinol, a considerable increase in the toxicity of the cytostatic drug occurs which may be fatal. The dosage of 6-MP or azathioprine should be reduced to a one-third or one-quarter dosage. Allopurinol inhibits the first-pass metabolism of orally administered 6-MP via xanthinoxidase.

Methotrexate

When administered at the same time as ASS, cotrimoxazole, penicillins and other NSARs, inhibition of the tubular secretion of MTX and the associated delay in elimination may lead to a considerable elevation in toxicity. This has also been described in individual case reports with respect to omeprazole.

Simultaneous administration should be avoided; patients receiving MTX should be interviewed following the use of these medications.

Paclitaxel

Paclitaxel is metabolized by CYP2C8 and CYP3A4. Paclitaxel is a substrate of p-glycoprotein.

Only a few studies concerning interactions exist. There are known interactions with ketoconazole as an enzyme inhibitor (efficacy is increased) and phenytoin as an inducer (efficacy is reduced). In general, interactions with other enzyme inhibitors or inducers are likely.

Case reports suggest that the plasma levels of doxorubicin and its active metabolite doxorubicinol are increased if administered in combination with paclitaxel. The most likely reason for this is the inhibition of CYP enzymes or p-glycoprotein by paclitaxel.

Teniposide

This is metabolized by CYP. Known interactions exist with phenytoin and phenobarbital, where a decrease in efficacy is observed.

Vinca alkaloids (vinblastine, vincristine, vinorelbine)

These are metabolized by CYP3A and are substrates of p-glycoprotein. Caution is therefore advised if administered simultaneously with inhibitors and inducers of these enzymes.

Vincristine

If administered in combination with CYP and p-glycoprotein inhibitor itraconazole, an increase in toxicity occurs. In individual case reports similar observations were reported for simultaneous administration with nifedipine.

If given at the same time as digoxin a decrease in the efficacy of the digoxin occurs due to vincristine interference with p-glycoprotein.

CONCLUSION

To date only a relatively small number of clinically relevant interactions with cytostatic drugs are known. However, it is assumed that numerous other such interactions exist. In general the use of these drugs in combination with a CYP or p-glycoprotein inducer or inhibitor is critical. Attention should be paid to indications of toxicity or loss of efficacy. Caution is also advised during the combined use with herbal medications, and certain nutritional components and supplements. In these cases patients should be interviewed regarding their use of these substances.

Knowledge and avoidance of clinically relevant interactions are vital aspects of ensuring quality in cytostatic drug therapy.

6
Measurement approaches of quality of life in oncology

S. SCHMIDT and M. BULLINGER

INTRODUCTION

The term 'health-related quality of life' has emerged in the medical field because of the recognition that long-term cancer treatment strongly affects multiple domains of life and therefore patient outcomes have to be given priority as an evaluation criterion for medical treatments. In the past three decades a range of activities have been initiated to develop outcome measures oriented at indicators of the quality of life rather than the quantity of life (e.g. ref. 1).

The need for psychometric methods to assess quality of life (QoL) has evolved, since traditional clinical parameters such as mortality or morbidity are limited in scope in explaining treatment outcomes in specific patient populations, and questions regarding the life situation of patients related to disease and therapy were much more relevant than before[2]. Changes in QoL might, for instance, be interpreted as an indicator of the impact of a new therapy, and also enhance the participation of patients into treatment[3].

The inclusion of the subjective perspective of patients has in no other field of psychosocial medicine been pursued so stringently and with such methodological rigor as in QoL research. Despite the moral impetus to include QoL measurement in oncology, and despite the vast amount of effort in instrument development, there are still a range of barriers towards implementing measures into clinical and research practice. This may be partly due to the confusion of how to use and interpret QoL in a variety of ways. The aim of this chapter is therefore to delineate the major approaches of QoL measurement after summarizing the state of the art of instrument development.

METHODS EMPLOYED IN QoL RESEARCH

There is a general consensus that the nature of QoL is both subjective and multidimensional[4]. Health-related QoL (HRQoL) has been defined as 'the extent to which one's usual or expected physical, emotional and social well-being are affected by a medical condition or its treatment'[5].

In QoL research a wide variety of psychometrically sound and normed measurement instruments are available on a national as well as an international level. It has been common to differentiate between disease-specific and generic measures of QoL[1].

Generic and disease-specific measures have both competing advantages and disadvantages, so their use is dependent on the aim of the investigation. In most cases it would be advisable to combine both assessment perspectives, because this provides both comparability across conditions and sensitivity towards treatment changes.

Disease-specific measures assess the specific impact of a condition on disease-related aspects of a patient's life, and can be employed to measure the impact of treatment in prospective studies with the sensitivity of the instrument being a major psychometric criterion. Generic measures can be employed in epidemiological surveys as well as in clinical studies with the aim of comparing different conditions in respect to their QoL.

Most measures, in particular generic measures, have been developed internationally in a psychometrically sound way, i.e. have been tested in respect to their reliability, validity and sensitivity. Some of the most common generic HRQoL measures are the SF-36 Health Survey[6,7], the Nottingham Health Profile[8] or the WHOQoL questionnaire[9]. One of the most common modular questionnaires is the EORTC questionnaire (= European Organisation for the Research and Treatment of Cancer[4]) for different types of cancer, which comprises generic as well as disease-specific scales, e.g. the BR23 module for breast cancer. Cella[5] provided a comprehensive overview of a broad range of QoL measures for patients with cancer, also recommending the use of measures which have been developed and/or extensively tested in cancer populations. Recent approaches in instrument development have also included focus group techniques in order to better capture the perspective of patients.

Depending on the approach of measurement, a difficult task is to identify a measure which could demonstrate a clear and significant contribution to care, which does not constitute a burden for the staff, which is perceived as unintrusive to patients and the treating staff and which nevertheless is appropriate for the aim of the investigation.

Along with the impetus to conduct online assessment of QoL, adaptive tests have been developed which construct the questionnaire at the time of assessment at the computer, thereby reducing the length of the questionnaire. These adaptive tests have been developed using modern psychometric methods. There are of course risks of using brief measures, and it should be taken into account whether to use a more aggregate or a more comprehensive scale, depending on the purpose of QoL assessment.

APPROACHES OF QoL MEASUREMENT

In the field of oncology, QoL has been included as a major outcome parameter because of its broad empirical basis and because of the plethora of measures and their potential use for clinical practice. Although quantifying treatment outcomes has often been the primary aim, there are a variety of potential applications of QoL research. In general, five broad approaches can be summarized, differing in the context, setting and aim of measurement.

1. Evaluative perspective. One of the major aims has been to evaluate the effect of treatments in the field of oncology, e.g. by comparing treatment groups in a prospective design. Two major methodological challenges have been discussed in this respect: (a) the problem of response shift which might occur in the course of treatment between two points of measurement and (b) the need to go beyond statistical significance and to question whether statistically significant changes are understandable and credible in the specific context and setting of assessment. Clinical significance questions whether statistically significant differences found in large samples are meaningful on a clinical level, or whether significant differences can be interpreted on the level of groups or individual scores. A variety of methodological approaches to estimate clinical significance have been developed[10,11].
2. Comparison of different clinical groups. The comparison of different patient populations, e.g. with different types of cancer, is one of the major aims in clinical studies. This might also take a range of socioeconomic, clinical and psychosocial determinants into account.
3. Prescriptive perspective. The use of QoL to estimate (health-care) needs of patients refers to the prescriptive potential of QoL measurement, but has been less frequently employed than clinical and intervention studies. QoL measure may be employed to estimate needs on a population basis, in clinical groups or even on individualized patients. The latter approach used in clinical practice has been separately summarized under the term 'integrated outcome measurement'.
4. Integrated, individualized outcome measurement. Only recently, QoL measurement has been used to assess individual patient profiles on a variety of QoL domains which may be implemented into routine clinical care.
5. Population-based approaches. The impairment of QoL of specific conditions can be compared both with other conditions and with an (age- and gender-appropriate) population level, e.g. by using population surveys.

In the following section we will provide an example for each of these measurement approaches.

Evaluation of treatment effects

One of the most frequently studied treatment modalities in QoL research has been the choice of the surgical method in patients with breast cancer[12,13]. Despite the considerable heterogeneity of empirical findings, a meta-analysis[14] identified modest advantages for breast-conserving therapy compared to mastectomy in the following psychosocial aspects: relationship satisfaction, sexuality, social adjustment, body and self image, as well as cancer-related fears and concerns. However, it was not possible to show in the majority of randomized controlled trials an effect of the surgical method on various aspects of quality of life (most frequently the two main operation methods, breast-conserving therapy and mastectomy were compared). Other factors which have been shown to influence the QoL outcome were the age of the patient (e.g. ref. 15), the stage of disease[16], specific surgical techniques[17], education and income level[18], and marital status, as well as both the setting and the timing of the QoL assessment. Former research suggests that breast cancer survivors obtain maximum recovery physically as well as psychologically 1 year after surgery[19]. However, women with greater mood disturbance and impaired body image 1 month after surgery, as well as lower income level and positive lymph nodes, displayed poorer outcome measures.

Comparison of different clinical groups

There is a variety of clinical studies including QoL outcomes comparing different types of cancer following a specific clinical focus. Most often these studies include further medical, psychosocial and sociodemographic determinants of QoL in order to gain a broader picture of the proportion of variance explained by different factors. As an example we describe a study comparing patients with invasive carcinoma and carcinoma *in situ*[30].

Preventive practice to screen for breast cancer and more effective treatment modes have led to a longer life expectancy of women; however, this also necessitates reflecting more strongly the emotional and physical consequences of the treatments and their side-effects[19]. In recent years the number of undetected carcinoma *in situ* as a pre-stage of breast cancer has increased.

Women diagnosed with a carcinoma *in situ* are in a particularly difficult situation since they are often confronted with the ambiguous position of being treated with a more radical form of surgery while being diagnosed with a non-invasive form of cancer. In this study a broad range of socioeconomic as well as psychosocial determinants were included because of their mediating effects in this specific clinical group.

Patients with carcinoma *in situ*, compared to patients diagnosed with an invasive type of cancer, displayed a higher QoL on various domains (see Figure 1); however, with coping strategies significantly mediating this relationship. In patients with carcinoma *in situ* there were strong tendencies to minimize the threat of cancer while patients with an invasive type of cancer used strategies oriented at seeking social support. In interpreting this finding the diverse clinical severity has to be taken into account. Concerning the participation of patients, patients with the *in situ* carcinoma reported more frequently that QoL aspects were considered by professionals and more frequently mentioned to be able to actively influence the course of treatment (see Figure 2).

A number of advantages might be assumed to integrate QoL at an early stage of disease. Clinical studies have shown:

1. that it enhances participation in the process of medical decision-making,
2. that the satisfaction with medical treatment is enhanced[20],
3. that the acceptance with the surgical choice is higher[21],
4. that perceived control and processing of the diagnosis are enhanced[22],
5. that the side-effects of affective disorders and emotional distress are reduced[23],
6. that communication of disease-related aspects with other family members is supported[21].

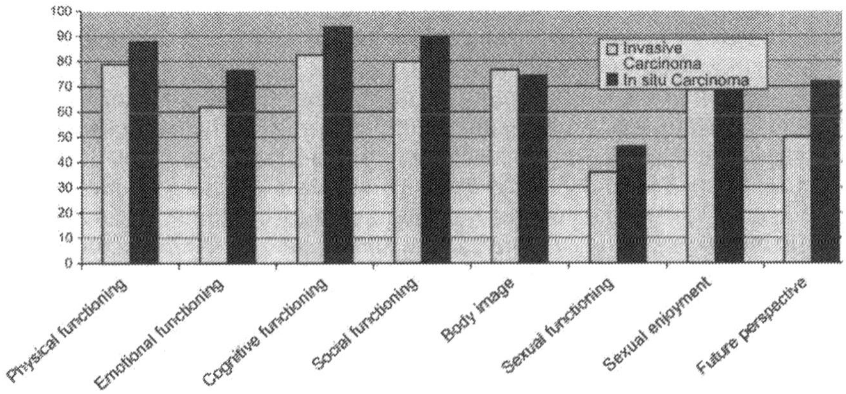

Figure 1 Comparison of QoL in patients with invasive breast cancer and carcinoma *in situ*

Prescriptive approaches

The prescriptive potential of QoL measurement is demonstrated in a field study on the quality of care in eastern Thuringia, Germany[25]. The aim of the prescriptive approach of QoL measurement is not only to highlight health-care needs in respect to medical treatment, but also to indicate areas for intervention to prevent serious emotional consequences of cancer, such as anxiety and depression.

In the Thuringia field study[25] it was possible to show that the need for intervention can be estimated on the basis of clinical and sociodemographic data. It was possible to identify subgroups on the basis of specific sociodemographic and clinical characteristics.

The QLQ30 and BR23 subgroups were characterized by outcome criteria obtained about 16 months after surgical treatment: side-effects, arm symptoms, breast symptoms, sexual functioning and future perspective analysis, which was strongly correlated with the QoL scales. The subgroups were characterized by:

1. multiple treatment-related side-effects and pessimism;
2. older, low scores of treatment-related side-effects, tendency to optimism;
3. average treatment related side-effects, tendency to pessimism;
4. younger patients with some treatment-related side-effects, optimism.

Both primary physical and psychological characteristics of a person were integrated into the approach. It was assumed that it was possible to use QoL scales, among others, as predictors for a successful intervention. These groups differed in the utilization of a rehabilitation programme, their motivation for this programme and their perceived success of this programme.

The first cluster was characterized by scores which indicate high intrusiveness of therapy modalities, low future perspective and sexual functioning. Women were highly educated, and often mentioned a worsening of their financial situation and self-esteem. In 36.4% of the cases the patients did not take part in a rehabilitation programme; but if they participated, there was a gain in knowledge as well as an improvement of their physical condition. In cluster one, low scores for future perspective and sexual functioning were associated with therapy-related side-effects. In these cases medical intervention programmes could be recommended to ease the symptoms.

Cluster 2 represents a subgroup of older women with low impact of side-effects as therapy-related symptoms and high scores of future perspective. The middle-range score for sexual functioning is related to the high rate of widowed women. When a rehabilitation programme was visited, a gain of knowledge was reported less often than an improvement in physical condition. According to the profile the necessitiy for an intervention appears not so obvious as for the other subgroups. However, an influence of social desirability cannot be ruled out with the applied instruments.

Cluster 3 is characterized by a psychic rather than physical intrusiveness. Thus although these women participated in rehabilitation programmes they often mentioned no notable benefit. For patients in cluster 3 it can be assumed that psychological support would reduce the intrusiveness of illness.

Cluster 4 is characterized by younger age with therapy-related symptoms, middle-range scores of future perspective and highest scores for sexual functioning. This group was also most frequently married (75%). The scores for future perspective were below average and the intrusiveness of operation-related interventions was high. A worsening of the financial situation appeared in 62.5% of cases. Although rehabilitation programmes were visited, a positive change of the physical condition was mentioned only 5.4% of the time, while increased knowledge regarding breast cancer was reported by 87.5% of the women.

While the approach of this study was to identify needs of larger clinical groups, the results initiated steps to implement QoL also on the basis of the individual patient.

Integrated, individualized outcome measurement

The prescriptive use of QoL indicators may be used on a population level; on the other hand its major purpose in clinical practice is a prescriptive indicator on an individual level in order to better adapt the provision of services to the individual needs of a patient. Individualized approaches of QoL assessment have only recently been introduced into medical care and may be characterized as a contribution to quality management in patient care. A prerequisite is to assess QoL by means of standardized questionnaires, and provide the technical opportunities to display the scales as QoL profiles which allow for a depiction of the individual case at a given time, as well as for the evaluation of the course of therapies. Adopting this methodological concept, a large field study involving practitioners aimed at researching therapy outcomes with regard to rectal and breast carcinoma[26]. Regular interim data analyses and discussion of the results in quality circle groups were used to improve the quality of care. Major challenges are a good timing of the assessment in the diagnostic process, a good graphical display and the commitment of medical doctors as well as nurses.

Population-related comparisons

Public health research has recently integrated QoL measures not only because of the purpose of describing the health status of a whole population but also to

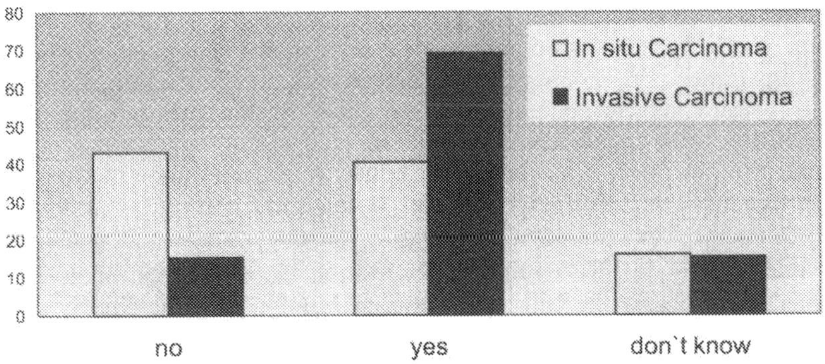

Figure 2 Percentage of perceived participation via QoL assessment in patients with breast cancer[30]

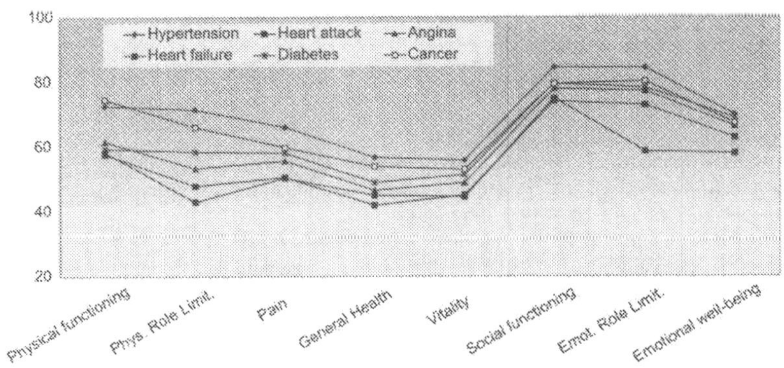

Figure 3 Quality of life profiles across various conditions, based on self report of a German health survey (higher scores indicate a better quality of life)[24]

compare different chronic conditions. For instance, the SF36 Health Survey has been normed and psychometrically tested in a German representative survey with a sample of 2013 persons. The German SF36 showed good psychometric properties while also showing age and gender effects. Since respondents also had to answer chronic conditions lists, it was possible to compare differential profiles of self-reported chronic conditions. Results show that HRQoL can provide a differentiated picture of various QoL domains, as suggested by the WHO definition.

The resulting SF36 scale profiles in general indicate a high, but a differential, impairment of individuals with chronic conditions, who do not show differential effects in the absolute impairment across different subscales (see Figure 3)[6]. It is noteworthy that QoL scale scores have been higher for patients with cancer (indicating less impairment) than in a range of other severe conditions, such as diabetes or coronary heart disease.

CONCLUSION

The aim of this chapter was not to provide a detailed and comprehensive account of QoL instruments in oncology, but to delineate the major existing approaches of QoL measurement in oncology, e.g. the public health approach, the clinical approach, the prescriptive approach and the ideographic approach oriented at optimizing routine care. It has been shown that QoL is not only a measure to be used in treatment-related studies, but can be interpreted from a variety of perspectives on the level of larger populations, clinical groups or the individual patient. The choice of the instruments, as well as the design and the interpretation of QoL measures, have to be appropriately attuned to the perspective and setting of QoL assessment.

References

1. Bowling A. Measuring Health: A Review of Quality of Life Measurement Scales. Philadelphia: Open University Press, 1991.
2. Bullinger M, Cella D, Anderson R, Aaronson NK. Creating and evaluating cross-national instruments. In: Spilker, B, editor. Quality of Life and Pharmaeconomics in Clinical Trials. Philadelphia: Lippincott-Raven, 1996;S659–68.
3. Cella D, Chang CH, Lai JS, Webster K. Advances in quality of life measurements in oncology patients. Semin Oncol. 2002;29(Suppl. 3): 60–8.
4. Aaronson NK, Ahmedzai S, Bergman B, Bullinger M. The European organization for research and treatment of cancer QLQ-C30: A quality-of-life instrument for use in international clinical trials in oncology. J Natl Cancer Inst. 1993;85:65–77.
5. Cella DF. Measuring quality of life in palliative care. Semin Oncol. 1995;22:73–81.
6. Bullinger M, Kirchberger I. SF-36 Fragebogen zum Gesundheitszustand. Göttingen: Hogrefe Verlag, 1998.
7. Ware JE, Sherbourne CD. The MOS 36-Item Short-Form Health Status Survey (SF-36): 1: conceptual framework and item selection. Med Care. 1992;30:473–83.
8. Hunt SM, McEwen J, McKenna SP et al. The Nottingham Health Profile: Subjective Health Status and Medical Consultations. Soc Sci Med. 1981;15A:221–9.
9. Power M, Bullinger M, Harper A, Group W. The World Health Organization WHOQOL-100: tests of the universality of quality of life in fifteen different cultural groups worldwide. Health Psychol. 1999;18:495–505.
10. Sloan JA, Cella D, Frost M, Guyatt GH, Sprangers M, Symonds T. Assessing clinical significance in measuring oncology patient quality of life: introduction to the symposium, content overview, and definition of terms. Mayo Clin Proc. 2002;77:367–70.
11. Cella D, Bullinger M, Scott C, Barofsky I. Group vs individual approaches to understanding the clinical significance of differences or changes in quality of life. May Clin Proc. 2002;77:384–92.
12. van Dongen JA, Voogd AC, Fentiman IS et al. Long-term results of a randomized trial comparing breast-conserving therapy with mastectomy: European Organization for Research and Treatment of Cancer. J Natl Cancer Inst. 2000;92:1143–50.
13. Veronesi U, Salvadori B, Luini A et al. Breast conservation is a safe method in patients with small breast cancer. Long term results of 3 randomized trials on 1,973 patients. Eur J Cancer. 1995; 31:1574–9.
14. Moyer A. Psychosocial outcomes of breast-conserving surgery versus mastectomy: a meta-analytic review. Health Psychol. 1997;16:284–98.
15. Wenzel, LB, Fairclough DL, Brady MJ et al. Age-related differences in the quality of life of breast cancer patients after treatment. Cancer. 1999;86:1768–74.
16. Hürny C, Bernhard J, Coates AS et al. Impact of adjuvant therapy on quality of life in women with node-positive operable breast cancer. International breast cancer study group. Lancet. 1996; 347:1279–84.
17. Maunsell E, Brisson C, Dubies L, Lauzier S, Fraser A. Work problems after breast cancer: an explanatory qualitative study. Psycho-Oncology. 1999;8:467–73.

18. Ganz PA, Schag AC, Lee J, Polinsky ML, Tan SJ. Breast conservation vs mastectomy. Is there a difference in psychological adjustment or quality of life in the year after surgery? Cancer. 1992; 68:1729–38.
19. Schnipper HH. Life after breast cancer. J Clin Oncol. 2001;19:3581–4.
20. Weiss SM, Wengert PA, Martinez EM, Sewall W, Kopp E. Patient satisfaction with decision-making for breast cancer therapy. Ann Surg Oncol. 1996;3:285–9.
21. Damian D, Tattersall MHN. Letters to patients: improving communication in cancer care. Lancet. 1991;338:923–5.
22. Fisher B, Britten N. Patient access to records: expectations of hospital doctors and experiences of cancer patients. Br J Gen Pract. 1993;43:52–6.
23. Johnson JA, Adelstein DJ. The use of recorded interviews to enhance physician patient communication. J Cancer Educ. 1991;6:99–102.
24. Bullinger M, Kirchberger I. SF-36 Fragebogen zum Gesundheitzustand. Göttingen: Hogrefe Verlag, 1998.
25. Nagel G, Schmidt S, Strauss B, Katenkamp D. Empirically derived subgroups of the EORTC-QLQ, BR 23 – a clinically oriented approach. Breast Cancer Res Treat. 2001;68:75–82.
26. Lorenz W, Koller M. Lebensqualitatsmessung als integraler Bestandteil des Qualitatsmanagements in der Operativen. Zentralbl Chir. 1996;121:545–51.
27. Aaronson NK. Assessing the quality of life of patients in cancer clinical trials: common problems and common sense solutions. Eur J Cancer. 1992;28A:1304–7.
28. Cella DF, Bonomi AE. Measuring quality of life. A 1995 update. Oncology. 1995;9:47–60.
29. Fallowfield L. Offering choice of surgical treatment to women with breast cancer. Patient Educ Counsel. 1997;30:209–14.
30. Jentschke TM. Bewältigungsprozesse bei Patientinnen mit In situ-Karzinomen: Ein Vergleich zur Bewältigung des Mammakarzinoms. Medizinische Dissertation, Universität Jena, 2002.
31. Kind P. The EuroQoL instrument: an index of health-related quality of life. In: Spilker B, editor. Quality of Life and Pharmaeconomics in Clinical Trials. Philadelphia: Lippincott-Raven, 1996: 191–202.
32. Kohlmann T, Bullinger M, Raspe HH. Die deutsche Form des Nottingham Health Profiles – Skalenstruktur, Reliabilität und Validität. Z Sozial- Präventivmedizin. 1997;42:175–85.
33. Soni MK, Cella, D. Quality of life and symptom measures in oncology: an overview. Am J Manag Care. 2002;8(Suppl. 18): S560–73.
34. Spilker B. Introduction to the field of quality of life trials. In: Spilker B, editor. Quality of Life and Pharmaeconomics in Clinical Trials. Philadelphia: Lippincott-Raven. 1996:S1–10.

Section III
Side-effects of chemotherapeutic agents: physiology, pathophysiology and terminology

7
Morphological changes of drug side-effects – view of the pathologist

Ch. WITTEKIND

INTRODUCTION

An increasing number of drugs affect the intestines and the liver. The mechanisms of damage may be unclear, but they can mimic a variety of other diseases. Different drugs act in different ways[1]. Mechanisms involved include direct damage to the lamina mucosa (physically), allergic reactions of varying intensity, influence on cell replication and apoptosis, initiation of an inflammatory response with accompanying reactions or damage of nerve plexus[1,2]. The main organs involved are the oesophagus, stomach, small and large intestine, and liver. Considering the multitude of damaging mechanisms, as well as the number of potentially damaging drugs, it is amazing that the frequency of drug-induced damage is rather low. In estimating the frequency of drug-induced damage a major problem is that the morphological effects of many clinically well-recognized drug-related diseases are often poorly documented and sometimes undocumented[2].

From a pathologist's point of view, with a few notable exceptions, most drug-associated diseases have no specific morphological features but tend to result in inflammation or ulceration. The diagnosis is therefore dependent initially on the suspicion that the clinical symptoms and morphological appearances may in some way be associated with a drug or medication which may not necessarily have been prescribed, but may have been obtained over the counter. The importance of a drug history and, if the pathologist is to be of any value at all, its availability to the pathologist, is apparent. Once suspected, the most important requirements are:

1. To establish temporal eligibility and confirm that the latent period between taking the drug and its adverse effect is reasonably consonant with past experience (if that exists). A time flow chart should be compiled, indicating the onset of symptoms and their relationship with the drug in question or with all drugs/medications that the patient has been using.

2. To link the suspected drug with markers such as exclusion, dechallenge, rechallenge, singularity of the drug, pattern (clinical, laboratory data, morphology), and quantitation or qualitation of the amount of the drug.
3. To ensure that the patient's new symptoms under investigation cannot be explained by the underlying disease or other associated diseases.
4. To estimate the certainty of the association (causative, probable, possible, coincidental, negative).

If the morphological features are not specific, as is frequently the case, it is often useful to consult a table of the causes of non-specific inflammation to ensure that the patient is not clearly predisposed to one of these on clinical grounds.

A general principle of drug-induced injury is that effects can be potentiated by a number of diseases of each particular organ. In this contribution the main mechanisms and morphological features of drug-induced damage in the organs mentioned above will be discussed.

IATROGENIC GASTROINTESTINAL ISCHAEMIA

The iatrogenic ischaemic disorders of the gastrointestinal tract are caused by drugs, trauma, and radiation injury[1,2]. Drugs-induced vascular disorders are listed in Table 1. Iatrogenic gastrointestinal ischaemia falls into two categories:

1. due to reduction in blood pressure, blood volume or both and
2. secondary to arterial obstruction or constriction.

Hypotensive and hypovolaemic agents causing non-occlusive vascular ischaemia are listed in Table 1. Many of the patients already have intrinsic vascular disease, and the drugs often merely contribute to the vascular insufficiency.

Table 1 Iatrogenic vascular disorders (adapted from ref. 2)

Drugs
Hypotensive and/or hypovolaemic agents
Diuretics, digoxin, reserpine, methyldopa
Catecholamines, ganglion blockers, alpha-adrenergic blockers
Antiarrhythmic drugs and some antidepressants
Thrombosis
Drug-induced vasculitis
Hypersensitivity vasculitis (e.g. allopurinol, indocin, ampicillin)
Toxic vasculitis (e.g. gold salts and sulphonamides)
Thrombocytopenia
Antineoplastic drugs
Thrombolytic agents
Anticoagulants (e.g. heparin, warfarin, coumadin)
Arterial spasm
Vasopressin
Ergot or derivatives
Methysergide maleate

Vascular obstruction or constriction can be due to thrombosis, vasculitis, or arterial spasm. There are two major causes of drug-induced arterial or venous thrombosis in the gastrointestinal tract, i.e. drug-induced hypercoagulable states and vasculitis.

Oestrogen medication and oral contraception are the major causes of the iatrogenic hypercoagulation disorders, and these may be potentiated by anticoagulants. These states can involve all vessels, including those of the gut, especially the superior mesenteric artery. There is evidence that the risk is related to the dosage of oestrogen. Smoking and hypertension are additional risk factors. On histological examination, in addition to finding recent thrombotic occlusion, there is frequently evidence of previous thrombosis characterized by focal marked intimal proliferation and an intact elastic lamina indicating absence of an underlying vasculitis.

Drug-induced vasculitis consists of two types: hypersensitivity and toxicity. Hypersensitivity forms of vasculitis may develop after the patient has been on drugs for months or years, or after a short interval following cessation of medication, for reasons that are unclear. A growing list of drugs have been implicated, including numerous antibiotics such as penicillins, tetracyclins, and chloramphenicol, the sulphonamides, allopurinol, diazepam, griseofulvin, indocin, isoniazid, spironolactone, and trimethadione. Histologically the lesions involve primarily arterioles, capillaries, and venules, with sparing of the larger vessels, and are characterized by a severe mononuclear infiltrate of the vessel wall and surrounding perivascular tissues, but without fibrinoid necrosis.

Toxic vasculitis involves primarily small and medium-sized arteries, although it may also involve arterioles, venules, and capillaries. Morphologically, it is similar to polyarteritis nodosa and results in similar complications. Causes of toxic vasculitis are non-protein drugs such as penicillins and sulphonamides.

Vasoconstrictor drugs, for example ergot, as in cafergot (an ergotamine–caffeine combination) and methysergide (used for migraine) have occasionally been reported to produce gastrointestinal ischaemia.

OESOPHAGUS

No characteristic pathological findings exist for drug-induced oesophagitis. Different drugs damage the oesophagus via different mechanisms. Age, posture, and dissolution pH of the medication influence drug-mediated oesophageal injury. Hiatal hernia, oesophageal dysmotility, or stricture predispose to prolonged retention and enhance the ability of drugs to damage the lamina mucosa[1].

Some injuries result from physical damage of the lamina mucosa. Other mechanisms are allergic in nature and may be suggested by the presence of eosinophilia in the absence of reflux disease. Some drugs directly damage replicating cells. Vincristine causes myenteric plexus damage and pseudo-obstruction syndromes. Drugs commonly involved in drug-induced oesophagitis include those listed in Table 2. Antibiotics account for at least half of the reported cases of drug-associated oesophagitis, with tetracycline being the commonest offender. The most dangerous drug-related oesophagitis results from potassium chloride[1].

Table 2 Drugs inducing oesophagitis (adapted from ref. 1)

Acetaminophen	Ibuprofen
Antimitotic agents	Indomethacin
Acelylsalicylic acid	Minocyclin
Ascorbic acid	Non-steroidal anti-inflammatory drugs
Barbiturates	Pantogar
Carbachol	Phenylbutazone
Chemotherapeutic agents	Phenobarbital
Chloral hydrate	Phenoxymethyl penicillin
Clindamycin	Potassium chloride
Cromolyn	Prednisone
Digoxin, digitoxin	Quinidine
Doxyclycine	Tetracycline
D-Penicillamine	Theophylline
Emepronium bromide	Tinidazole
Erythromycin	Tolectin
Ferrous salts	Zidovudine (AZT)

Table 3 Morphological changes of drug-associated damage in the oesophagus

Epithelial lesions
Subepithelial oedema
Basal cell hyperplasia
Thickening of the stratum corneum
Presence of balloon cells
Mild atypia
Numerous mitoses

The morphological changes associated with drug injury are listed in Table 3. None of them can be considered specific either for a drug injury or for a specific drug.

STOMACH

Side-effects of many drugs may be encountered in the stomach, mostly gastric erosions, haemorrhage, and necrosis. Some drug-induced and stress-induced ulcers share common cellular pathogenetic events, but the factors that lead to the initial cellular damage may differ. Non-steroidal anti-inflammatory drugs (NSAIDs) represent the commonest cause of macroscopic gastric injury and the most severe side-effects in the United States. Histologically, an inflammatory reaction is not very pronounced, with some changes indicating a drug injury; these are listed in Table 4. The most frequent morphological changes are subepithelial haemorrhages, erosions, and ulcers. It is important to recognize that NSAID-associated erosions and subepithelial haemorrhages occur soon after NSAID ingestion, that adaptation takes place in time, and that they are located in both the body and antrum, whereas NSAID-associated ulcers dominate in the antrum and, to a lesser extent, in the duodenum. NSAIDs produce mucosal injury via local and systemic effects[3,4]. Recently it was postulated that the histology of necrosis in the stomach mucosa may indicate the reason for the

Table 4 Clues that suggest the presence of chemical injury of stomach (adapted from ref. 1)

Pit expansion
Mucus depletion
Superficial oedema
No organisms present
No metaplasia
No polyps
No enlarged folds
Muscle fibres extending into the mucosa from the muscularis mucosae
Villiform transformation

Table 5 Drugs inducing damage in stomach

Non-steroidal anti-inflammatory drugs (NSAIDs)
aspirin
Steroids
Chemotherapy
H_2 receptor antagonists
Prostaglandin therapy
Cocaine use
Alcohol

damage, e.g. NSAID-associated versus *Helicobacter pylori*-associated[5]. Aspirin is the best-studied NSAID, but it appears that the mechanisms of injury with other NSAIDs are similar to those of aspirin. A major systemic mechanism is inhibition of prostaglandin synthesis via inhibition of cyclooxygenase[3]. Aspirin also changes the ability of the mucosa to maintain a pH gradient, and results in the phenomenon of back-diffusion of gastric acid with resultant mucosal injury. The effects of aspirin are more pronounced in older than in younger patients. Subepithelial haemorrhages and erosions have been documented in volunteers given oral iron. Hepatic arterial chemotherapy can produce gastric erosions and large ulcers. Drugs inducing injury in the stomach are listed in Table 5.

LARGE BOWEL

We know a large variety of changes in the large bowel are caused by drug injury[2]. As discussed above, ischaemic injury of the bowel is frequently multi-factorial. Some drug effects are listed in Table 6. Besides these drugs there are some more which can cause an inflammation similar to that which can be observed in inflammatory bowel disease, ischaemic or infectious colitis. This group of drugs comprises sulphasalazine, alpha-methyl-dopa and penicillamine[6].

NSAIDs cause a spectrum of diseases affecting the gastrointestinal tract. NSAID-associated large intestinal disease is probably an underdiagnosed entity. In one study, in which Crohn's colitis had been excluded, four of 43 new cases of colitis were thought to be based on NSAIDs[6]. The described histology suggests an increase in lymphocytes and particularly plasma cells with occasional crypt abscesses and even occasional giant cells but no granulomas. There is little or no

Table 6 Effects of drugs in colon and rectum (adapted from ref. 2)

Laxatives abuse	Pseudomelanosis coli, neuromuscular injury
Anticholinergics	
Antidepressives	
Chemotherapeutic drugs	Decreased mitotic activity, cell death
	Induction of apoptosis, cell death
Tranquillizers	Injury to myenteric plexus
Various drugs	Pseudo-obstruction
Alcohol	
Clonidine	
Cimetidine	
Loperamide	
NSAIDs	Colitis, ulcers, haemorrhages, perforation, strictures
Heavy metal	
Arsenic	
Quicksilver	Enterocolitis
Silver	Pain, fever, proteinuria, skin changes
Antibiotics	Pseudomembranous colitis
Alpha-interferon	Vasculitis

architectural distortion. If acute inflammation or ulceration is present it is usually superficial, with a luminal neutrophilic infiltrate reminiscent of a pseudomembrane but without the mucus, epithelium, or red blood cells.

The microscopic appearance of gold-associated colitis varies from a mucosa that is completely ulcerated and includes pseudomembranous changes to one which regenerates with relatively few crypts[7].

Laxatives fall into several distinct categories and act by a variety of mechanisms. Although only pseudomelanosis is readily recognized histologically, electron microscopic observations of patients with chronic laxative abuse have shown damage to the microvilli, reduction of and abnormalities in cytoplasmic organelles, and an increase in the number of lysozymes and dense bodies[8]. The dirty-brown, occasionally almost black, lipofuscin-like pigment is found in macrophages in the lamina propria. Surprisingly, the pigment is easily missed when present only in small quantities, because macrophages need to be deliberately sought out and examined for the presence of pigment[2]. The action of anthraquinones is not only exerted on the mucosa but causes considerable damage to the myenteric plexus, with loss of neurons and schwannosis.

Antineoplastic and immunosuppressive agents have direct effects on the gut, initially causing mitotic arrest. This may result in necrosis of the mucosa. Initially the mucosa architecture may be preserved, but with an excess of pyknotic nuclei which have been called apoptotic bodies; they are found particularly near the crypt base. Combination chemotherapy induces more marked effects. A characteristic feature of chemotherapy seems to be the focal variation of the damage even from crypt to crypt, some crypts being relatively severely damaged while adjacent ones remain relatively unaffected[2].

Alcohol is reported to cause a reduction in the number of goblet cells in rectal mucosa; a chronic inflammatory infiltrate has also been described.

LIVER

Many chemical agents (about 1000 drugs) can produce hepatic injury. The relative importance of hepatic injury due to various types of exposure to toxins has changed considerably over the years. To most clinicians and pathologists, hepatic injury caused by adverse reactions to medical agents is more important than that caused by other substances. Nevertheless, adverse reactions to drugs have ranked numerically as a relatively minor cause of acute hepatic disease. Less than 5% of instances of jaundice in several series have been attributed to drug reactions[9,10]. However, subsequent analyses suggested that 10% of cases of apparent 'hepatitis' are due to drug-induced injury, the figure rising to over 40% in patients above the age of 50. Up to 25% of cases of fulminant hepatic failure may be the result of adverse reactions to medical agents[11,12]. Drug-induced cholestasis appears to outrank other causes of acute cholestasis[13].

There are two main categories of agents that can produce hepatic injury (Table 7). One consists of intrinsic hepatotoxins, i.e. they are predictable or true hepatotoxins (experimentally reproducible, dose-dependent); the others are idiosyncratic (facultative, non-predictable, non-dose-dependent), and they produce hepatic injury in the small proportion of exposed individuals who are unusually susceptible.

The main types of morphological changes in the liver produced by drugs are listed in Table 8. Definition of the forms of injury produced by the hepatotoxins

Table 7 Classification of hepatotoxic agents and major characteristics of each group (adapted from ref. 18)

Category of agent	*Incidence*	*Experimental reproducibility*	*Dose-dependence*	*Mechanism*	*Histology*	*Examples*
Intrinsic toxicity						
Direct				Direct physicochemical destruction by peroxidation of:		
Cytotoxic	High	Yes	Yes	hepatocytes	Necrosis/ steatosis	CCl_4
Cholestatic	High	Yes	Yes	ductal cells	Cholestasis, duct destruction	Paraquat
Indirect				Interference with specific pathways or selective lesions in:		
Cytotoxic	High	Yes	Yes	hepatocytes	Necrosis Steatosis	
Cholestatic	High	Yes	Yes	ductal cells	Cholestasis Duct destruction	
Host idiosyncrasy						
Immunological (hypersensitivity)	Low	No	No	Drug allergy	Necrosis or cholestasis	Phenytoin, halothane
Metabolic	Low	No	No	Production of hepatotoxic metabolites	Necrosis or cholestasis	Isoniazid

Table 8 Morphological types of drug injury

Type of injury	*Agent (comment)*
Acute	
Cytotoxic	
Necrosis	
Zonal	
Perivenular	CCl_4, acetaminophen, halothane
Mid	Furusemide
Periportal	Allylformate, albitocin
Massive	Trinitrotoluene, some other drugs
Diffuse (panacinar)	Some drugs
Focal	Some drugs
Spotty	Some drugs
Apoptosis	Large number of agents
Steatosis	
Microvesicular	Ethionine, tetracycline, ethanol
Macrovesicular	Ethanol, methotrexate
Cholestatic	
Hepatocanalicular	Erythromycin, organic arsenicals
Canalicular	Contraceptive steroids
Vascular	
Hepatic vein injury	Antineoplastic agents
Peliosis hepatis	Medroxyprogesterone
Hepatic vein thrombosis	Contraceptive steroids
Chronic	
Parenchymal	Oxyphenisatin, methyldopa, nitrafurantoin, clometacine, sulphonamide, ethanol, antineoplastic agents
Cholestatic	Haloperidol, imipramine, thiobendazole, tolbutamide
Vascular	Antineoplastic agents, and many others
Granulomas	Many drugs
Neoplasms	
Adenoma, hepatocellular	Contraceptive steroids, anabolic steroids
Carcinoma, hepatocellular or cholangiocarcinoma	Anabolic steroids, vinyl chloride
Angiosarcoma	Vinyl chloride, anabolic steroids

has been relatively simple, since the hepatic damage can be reproduced in experimental animals. Characterization of the forms of idiosyncratic injury, however, has been more difficult, and has depended on collation of materials from reports of individuals and groups of cases. However, histological changes are not typical for different drugs but only a sign. In differential diagnosis they should be considered against a multitude of other liver-damaging diseases.

Necrosis, degeneration and steatosis of hepatocytes can occur in various combinations. Indeed, toxic hepatic damage can cause virtually all of the morphological lesions known in hepatology. Necrosis can be subdivided into non-zonal necrosis and zonal necrosis (Table 8). Degeneration of hepatocytes precedes necrosis. A typical form of degeneration of hepatocytes (hyaline type) is the Mallory body, seen in alcoholic liver disease and a number of other diseases. Fatty degeneration (steatosis) can be produced by a large number of agents.

Two main types of steatosis occur – macrovesicular and microvesicular – the latter generally being acute. Necrosis induced by most drugs is accompanied by relatively slight inflammation. In general it appears to be less prominent than the inflammatory response to necrosis of equal severity caused by viral hepatitis. An exception is the injuries caused by phenytoin and para-aminosalicylic acid, which usually lead to a striking infiltration of mononuclear cells with or without eosinophils[14].

Some agents lead to injury that appears to spare the parenchyma and to cause only or mainly arrested bile flow. The histological manifestation of cholestatic injury consists mainly of bile accumulation in the cytoplasm of hepatocytes, and of bile casts in canaliculi and, at times, in cholangioles. Some agents cause minor cholestatic damage and rather a portal inflammatory reaction sometimes accompanied by destruction of ducts (e.g. paraquat poisoning)[13,15,16]. Some drugs produce a mixed form of hepatic injury, both hepatocellular and cholestatic (e.g. phenytoin)[7,17,18].

Chronic hepatic injury can manifest itself as chronic hepatitis, fibrosis, rarely cirrhosis, chronic cholestatic lesions, vascular lesions, and neoplasms[19–21].

Other drug-associated morphological changes consist of subcapsular haematoma (e.g. oral anticoagulants), adaptive changes such as ground-glass hepatocytes (e.g. disulphiram), pigment deposits such as lipofuscin, black pigment, and haemosiderin, to name but a few.

Several risk factors may modify the effects of drugs: age, gender, malnutrition, obesity, diabetes mellitus, pre-existing liver disease, kidney diseases, cardiovascular diseases, psoriasis, pregnancy, AIDS, polychemotherapy, radiation therapy, etc.

References

1. Fenoglio-Preiser CM, Noffsinger AE, Stemmermann GN, Lantz PE, Listrom MB Rilke FO. Gastrointestinal Pathology. An Atlas and Text. Philadelphia: Lippincott-Raven, 1999:31–91.
2. Lewin KJ, Riddell RH, Weinstein WM. Drug-associated diseases of the small and large intestine. In: Lewin KJ, Riddell RH, Weinstein WM, editors. Gastrointestinal Pathology and its Clinical Implications. New York: Igaku-Shoin, 1992:1087–112.
3. Soll AH (Moderator). Non-steroidal anti-inflammatory drugs and peptic ulcer. Ann Intern Med. 1991;114:307–19.
4. Szabo S, Spill WF, Rainsford KD. Non-steroidal anti-inflammatory drug-induced gastropathy. Mechanisms and management. Med Toxicol Advers Drug Exp. 1989;4:77–94.
5. Vieth M, Müller H, Stolte M. Can the diagnosis of NSAID-induced or Hp-associated gastric ulceration be predicted from histology? Z Gastroenterol. 2002;40:783–8.
6. Tanner AR, Raghunath AS. Colonic inflammation and non-steroidal anti-inflammatory drug administration. An assessment of the frequency of the problem. Digestion. 1988;41:116–20.
7. Riddell RH. The gastrointestinal tract. In: Riddell RH, editor. The Pathology of Drug-induced and Toxic Diseases. New York: Churchill Livingstone, 1982:515–606.
8. Riemann JF, Schenk J, Ehler E et al. Ultrastructural changes of colonic mucosa in patients with chronic laxative abuse. Acta Hepatogastroenterol. 1978;25:213–18.
9. Bjornoboe M, Iversen O, Olsen S. Infective hepatitis and toxic jaundice in a municipal hospital during a five-year period. Acta Med Scand. 1967;182:491–501.
10. Koff RS, Gardner P, Harinasuta U, Phil CO. Profile of hyperbilirubinaemia in three hospital populations. Clin Res. 1970;18:680–1.
11. Hoofnagle JH, Carithers RL, Shapiro C, Ascher N. Fulminant hepatic failure: summary of a workshop. Hepatology. 1999;21:240–51.

12. Trey C, Lipworth L, Chalmers T et al. Fulminant hepatic failure. Presumable contribution of halothane. N Engl J Med. 1968;333:1118–27.
13. Zimmerman HJ, Lewis JH. Drug induced cholestasis. Med Toxicol. 1987;2:112–60.
14. Ishak KG, Zimmerman HJ. Morphologic spectrum of drug-induced hepatic disease. Gastroenterol Clin N Am. 1995:24:759–86.
15. Zimmerman HJ, Ishak KG. General aspects of drug-induced liver disease. Gastroenterol Clin N Am. 1995;24:739–57.
16. Zimmerman HJ. Hepatotoxicity. The Adverse Effects of Drugs and Other Chemicals to the Liver. Philadelphia: Lippincott Williams & Williams, 1999.
17. Mayoral W, Lewis JH, Zimmerman HJ. Drug-induced liver disease. Curr Opin Gastroenterol. 1999;15:208–16.
18. Zimmerman HJ, Ishak KG. Hepatic injury due to drugs and toxins. In: MacSween RNM, Burt AD, Portmann B, Ishak KG, Scheuer PJ, Anthony PP, editors. Pathology of the Liver, 4th edn. London: Churchill Livingstone, 2002:621–709.
19. Mays ET, Christofferson W. Hepatic tumours induced by sex steroids. Semin Liver Dis. 1984; 4:147–58.
20. Teschke R. Arzeimittelbedingte Lebererkrankungen. Z Gastroenterol. 2002;40:305–26.
21. Teschke R. Leberschäden durch Arzneimittel. Dtsch Med Wochenschr. 2002;127:1953–7.

8
Cell cycle of the mucosa and gland organs of the gastrointestinal system – physiology and influence of chemotherapeutic agents

J. SIEBLER and P. R. GALLE

INTRODUCTION

Mucosal cell proliferation is essential for the maintenance of the integrity of the gastrointestinal system. The proliferation rates of the gastrointestinal tract are high, so many cytotoxic agents of therapeutic interest are dose-limited because of gastrointestinal side-effects. Any part of the gastrointestinal tract can be affected, resulting in dysphagia, dyspepsia, malabsorption and diarrhoea. The routine assessment of gastrointestinal toxicity of chemotherapy is based on the patient's symptoms. The severity of stomatitis and frequency of diarrhoea are the commonly used criteria for grading gastrointestinal toxicity. The degree of involvement of the oral mucosa may not reflect the extent of the mucositis in distal locations. The frequency of diarrhoea may be affected by additional factors associated with nutrition, microbial environment or involvement of the gastrointestinal tract by the tumour.

For understanding the gastrointestinal side-effects of cytotoxic agents it is important to know some indications of the interference of these agents on the cell cycle. Most cytotoxic agents act on proliferating cells at a particular phase of their cell cycle. Apart from their direct inhibiting effect on cell division, the most frequent mode of cell death in consequence of chemotherapeutics is apoptosis. Among the repertoire of cellular responses to stress, the tumour suppressor protein p53 has been shown to play a critical role in determining the fate of cells with genomic damage. Here we summarize aspects of cell cycle regulation and the interference of 5-FU and CPT-11 (irinotecan).

CELL CYCLE AND CELL PROLIFERATION

Cell migration, cell kinetic and regeneration studies of the gastrointestinal mucosa have shown that cells derive from a relatively small number of stem cells. These stem cells are located at or near the base of the crypts[1]. Their position can be identified by counting cell positions from the base of the crypt. There are no biochemical or molecular markers for intestinal stem cells. Daughter cells differentiate in four cell lineages: absorptive enterocytes, comprising 80% of all epithelial cells; goblet cells; enteroendocrine cells; and Paneth cells. As cells exit the crypt onto the villus they stop cycling and go into the G1 phase of the cell cycle as a result of down-regulation of cyclin D1 and cyclin-dependent kinase 2[2]. While migrating up the crypt they continue to differentiate and, after 2–3 days, they reach the villus tip. In the mouse they are shed at a rate of 1400 cells/villus every 24 h. Thus the intestinal epithelium has one of the most rapid turnover rates among mammalian tissues. The process of cell division is divided into four different phases. The mitosis or M phase of the cell cycle can easily be recognized, because chromosomes are distributed among daughter cells. Then the cells enter a stage called G(ap)1, which is the most variable phase in duration. The next phase of the cell cycle is the S phase, in which DNA synthesis occurs. Immediately before mitosis cells enter a short, second gap phase, G2, where the cells prepare for mitosis and assemble the spindle proteins. The duration of the cell cycle is mainly determined by the length of the G1 phase, while the other phases are relatively constant. There is great variability in the length of the G1 phase in different tissues, so it seems to be a key element in controlling the cell cycle. Within the G1 phase the decision is made as to whether the cell leaves the cell cycle and differentiates or enters a resting phase called G0. Intracellular or extracellular events which influence the cell cycle progression act on critical control points or 'checkpoints', G1/S and G2/M[3,4]. One of the most important control proteins of the G1/S checkpoint is the retinoblastoma protein pRB regulated by multicomponent pathways and interplay between D-type cyclins, cyclin-dependent kinase (CDK) inhibitors and the p19ARF-mdm2-p53-pathway. The phosphorylation of pRB is necessary to overcome the checkpoint and to induce genes for DNA replication[5]. Cyclins and CDK are cell cycle regulators critical for error-free execution of these events. Many extracellular signals such as cytokines influence the progression of the cell cycle; for example growth factors cause cells in G0 phase to enter and proceed through the cycle. DNA damage activitates the G1/S checkpoint and the G2/M checkpoint. Consistent with their positive versus negative effects on cell cycle progression, the G1/S regulators qualify as either proto-oncogenes (e.g. cyclins D1, D2 and E) or tumour suppressors (p16, $p21^{Waf1/Cip1}$, pRB). Each of these proteins may become deregulated via several distinct molecular mechanisms[6]. Control of the G2/M checkpoint has been intensively studied in yeast[7]. Several genes such as rad9, rad17, mec1, mec2, and mec3 are activated by DNA damage, resulting in G2 arrest. Little is known regarding control in mammalian cells; G2 arrest seems to be regulated in part by the ataxia–telangiectasia–mutated (ATM) gene product. Deregulated cell proliferation, together with suppressed apoptosis, build the minimal common platform for the initiation of tumour growth.

INFLUENCE OF CHEMOTHERAPEUTIC AGENTS ON THE CELL CYCLE

Cytotoxic drugs and chemicals initiate apoptosis in intestinal epithelia after administration *in vivo*[8]. Stem cells in the small intestine were largely spared, and rapidly dividing early transit cells underwent frequent apoptosis[9].

The 'classic' view of drug toxicity is based on the drug–target interaction and its relation to a distinct cell cycle phase. For example, pharmacological S-phase synchronization was thought to sensitize tumour cells to anticancer drugs most toxic to DNA synthesis[10,11]. Apoptosis links the cell cycle phase preference of cytotoxic agents to the DNA damage checkpoint-initiated cell death programme. In the case of an intact checkpoint control, drug-mediated cell death is now understood as checkpoint response to DNA damage. The acuteness and severity of drug-induced DNA damage are not only related to the drug–target interaction, but also depend on the dose and time of application. While low doses leading to minor, repairable damage may only delay cell cycle progression, higher doses resulting in severe DNA damage initiate apoptosis or necrosis. Epithelial injury may occur throughout the gastrointestinal tract and cause mucositis, pharyngitis, dysphasia, oesophagitis, gastritis, colitis, or proctitis. Watery or bloody diarrhoea can lead to dehydration and hypotension. Supportive care with antidiarrhoeal agents such as loperamide, and sufficient hydration should be given if diarrhoea occurs. If the granulocyte nadir coincides with diarrhoea there is an increased risk of overwhelming sepsis.

One of the most common treatments in combination with other agents is 5-fluorouracil (5-FU). Oral and intestinal mucositis with diarrhoea has been shown to be the most frequent problem after the application of 5-FU, and its gastrointestinal toxicity is the main and dose-limiting side-effect. 5-FU cytotoxicity depends on conversion to nucleotides 5-fluoro-UTP, 5-fluoro-dUMP, and 5-fluoro-dUTP. These metabolites can act in a number of ways to induce cytotoxicity. Binding of 5-fluoro-dUMP to the enzyme inhibitor thymidilate synthase inhibits the synthesis of thymidine nucleotides. Inhibition of thymidilate synthase leads to DNA strand breaks, believed to be the result of ribosylthymine 5′-triphosphate depletion and probably misincorporation of dUTP into DNA[12]. There is also an incorporation of UTP into RNA which interferes with normal RNA processing and function. The extent of 5-FU-RNA incorporation correlates with cytotoxicity in tissue culture and *in vivo* models[13,14]. DNA damage is sensed by kinases such as the DNA-dependent protein kinase (DNA-PK) or ATM-kinase leading to phosphorylation and activation of p53[15–17]. p53 transmits the apoptotic signal by a complicated mechanism that involves its ability to transactivate a series of p53-inducible genes[18,19]. This results in cell cycle arrest or activation of apoptosis pathways. Müller et al.[20] showed that p53 induces the transcription of the CD95 gene in response to DNA damage by 5-FU and other anticancer drugs. The activation of $p21^{Waf1/Cip1}$ induced by p53 leads to an inhibition of cyclinE/cdk2 activity which prevents phosphorylation of pRB. This results in cell cycle G1 arrest[21]. Without functional $p21^{Waf1/Cip1}$ cells fail to arrest the cell cycle. Apart from induction of cell cycle arrest or apoptosis p53 is also involved in DNA repair; for example, fibroblasts homozygous for mutant p53 are deficient in global DNA repair[22,23]. Tanaka et al.[24] described a p53-inducible gene, p53R2, encoding a a ribonucleotide reductase that is directly involved in the p53 checkpoint for repair of DNA damage.

The important role of p53 for the development of 5-FU-induced diarrhoea was elucidated by $p53^{-/-}$ mice. These mice showed significantly less histopathological intestinal damage than their wild-type counterparts 72–96 h after the administration of two doses of 400 mg/kg 5-FU[25]. However, this effect is not simply a reflection of the p53-null mice showing less apoptosis, but additionally resulted from the lack of p53-dependent inhibition of cell cycle progression.

Another group of cytotoxic agents frequently used in treatment of gastrointestinal cancer are the topoisomerase inhibitors. Topoisomerases are nuclear enzymes essential for DNA replication, RNA transcription, chromosomal condensation and mitotic chromatid separation[26]. The level of topoisomerase I is independent of cell cycle phases although cytotoxicity is manifest only in proliferating cells. Topoisomerase II is cell cycle phase dependent, being absent in the G0/G1 phase with an increase at the onset of the S phase and during the G2 phase of the cell cycle[27]. The topoisomerase active agents currently in clinical use stabilize a transient covalent enzyme–DNA complex, which produces DNA strand cleavage and leads to cell death by apoptosis[28]. The topoisomerase I-inhibitor irinotecan (CPT-11) is enzymatically activated to the metabolite SN-38. The most frequent side-effect is diarrhoea in more than 70%. CPT-11 is also associated with a higher risk of severe diarrhoea grade III–IV, according to the NCI/WHO common toxicity criteria[29]. Mice treated with irinotecan exhibited intestinal wall thinning with epithelial vacuolation, vascular dilatation, inflammatory cell infiltrate and evidence of apoptosis[30]. CPT-11 induces early diarrhoea with cholinergic syndrome within the first 24 h of administration and it is also responsible for a late diarrhoea occurring more than 24 h after CPT-11 infusion. The early diarrhoea is caused by mimicking the effects of acetylcholine so in both animal models and humans the symptoms are inhibited by administration of the anticholinergic drug atropine[31]. The late diarrhoea is propably induced by direct damage to the intestinal epithelium resulting in a leaky mucosa unable to absorb fluid and an increase of secretion of fluid by the intestinal epithelium[32].

Because chemotherapy and radiation therapy for cancer often have severe side-effects limiting their efficacy, strategies should be developed to prevent damage to normal tissues. p53 is a key component of the cellular emergency response mechanism, and its lack is accompanied by high rates of genomic instability, rapid tumour progression, resistance to anticancer therapy and increased angiogenesis. However, p53 is also involved in chemotherapy-induced side-effects; for example, p53-dependent apoptosis occurs in sensitive tissues shortly after gamma irradiation and p53-deficient mice survive higher doses of gamma irradiation than wild-type mice[33,34]. Komarov et al.[35] showed that the chemical inhibitor of p53, pifithrin-α, protected mice from side-effects of cancer therapy. In addition to the development of chemotherapeutic agents more specific to tumour cells, these results may contribute towards detecting and creating substances diminishing the side-effects of cytotoxic agents.

References

1. Potten CS, Booth C, Pritchard DM. The intestinal epithelial stem cell: the mucosal governor. Int J Exp Pathol. 1997;78:219–43.
2. Chandrasekaran C, Coopersmith CM, Gordon JI. Use of normal and transgenic mice to examine the relationship between terminal differentiation of intestinal epithelial cells and accumulation of their cycle regulators. J Biol Chem. 1996;271:28414–21.
3. Elledge SJ. Cell cycle checkpoints: preventing an identity crisis. Science. 1996;274:1664–72.
4. McDonald ER 3rd, El-Deiry WS. Checkpoint genes in cancer. Ann Med. 2001;33:113–22.
5. Dulic V, Kaufmann WK, Wilson SJ et al. p53-dependent inhibition of cyclin-dependent kinase activities in human fibroblasts during radiation-induced G1 arrest. Cell. 1994;76:1013–23.
6. Hall M, Peters G. Genetic alteration of cyclins, cyclin-dependent kinases, and Cdk inhibitors in human cancer. Adv Cancer Res. 1996;68:67–108.
7. Hartwell LH, Kastan MB. Cell cycle control and cancer. Science. 1994;266:1821–8.
8. Ijiri K, Potten CS. Response of intestinal cells of differing topographical and hierarchical status to ten cytotoxic drugs and five sources of radiation. Br J Cancer. 1983;47:175–85.
9. Ijiri K, Potten CS. Further studies on the response of intestinal crypt cells of different hierarchical status to eighteen different cytotoxic agents. Br J Cancer. 1987;55:113–23.
10. Del Bino G, Lassota P, Darzynkiewicz Z. The S-phase cytotoxicity of camptothecin. Exp Cell Res. 1991;193:27–35.
11. Erba E, Len S, Lorico A, D'Incaci M. Potentiation of etoposide cytotoxicity against a human ovarian cancer cell line by pretreatment with non-toxic concentrations of methotrexate or aphidicolin. Eur J Cancer. 1992;28:66–71.
12. Curtin N, Harris A, Aherne G. Mechanism of cell death following thymidylate synthase inhibition: 2′-deoxyuridine-5′-triphosphate accumulation, DNA damage, and growth inhibition following exposure to CB3717 and dipyridamole. Cancer Res. 1991;51:2346–52.
13. Kufe DW, Major PP. 5-Flurouracil incorporation into human breast carcinoma RNA correlates with cytotoxicity. J Biol Chem. 1981;256:9802.
14. Glazer RI, Loyd LS. Association of cell lethality with incorporation of 5-fluorouracil and 5-fluorouridine into nuclear RNA in human colon carcinoma cell culture. Mol Pharmacol. 1982;21:468.
15. Siciliano JD, Camman CE, Taya Y, Sakaguchi K, Apella E, Kastan MB. DNA damage induces phosphorylation of the amino terminus of p53. Genes Dev. 1997;11:3471–81.
16. Pritchard DM, Watson AJ, Potten CS, Jackman AL, Hickman JA. Inhibition by uridine but not thymidine of p53-dependent intestinal apoptosis initiated by 5-fluorouracil: evidence for the involvement of RNA pertubation. Proc Natl Acad Sci USA. 1997;94:1795–9.
17. Woo RA, McLure KG, Lees-Miller SP, Rancourt DE, Lee PW. DNA-dependent protein kinase acts upstream of p53 in response to DNA damage. Nature. 1998;394:700–4.
18. Miyashita T, Reed JC. Tumor suppressor p53 is a direct transcriptional activator of the human bax gene. Cell. 1995;80:293–9.
19. Polyak K, Xia Y, Zweier JL, Kinzler KW, Vogelstein B. A model for p53 induced apoptosis. Nature. 1997;389:300–5.
20. Müller M, Wilder S, Bannasch D et al. p53 activates the CD95 (APO-1/Fas) gene in response to DNA damage by anticancer drugs. J Exp Med. 1998;188:2033–45.
21. el-Deiry WS, Harper JW, O'Connor PM et al. WAF1/CIP1 is induced in p53-mediated G1 arrest and apoptosis. Cancer Res. 1994;54:1169–74.
22. Deng C, Zhang P, Harper JW, Elledge SJ, Leder P. Mice lacking p21CIP1/WAF1 undergo normal development, but are defective in G1 checkpoint control. Cell. 1995;82:675–84.
23. Brugarolas J, Chandrasekaran C, Gordon JI, Beach D, Jacks T, Hannon GJ. Radiation-induced cell cycle arrest compromised by p21 deficiency. Nature. 1995;377:552–7.
24. Tanaka H, Arakawa H, Yamaguchi T et al. A ribonucleotide reductase gene involved in a p53-dependent cell-cycle checkpoint for DNA damage. Nature. 2000;404:42–9.
25. Pritchard DM, Potten CS, Hickman JA. The relationships between p53-dependent apoptosis, inhibition of proliferation, and 5-fluorouracil-induced histopathology in murine intestinal epithelia. Cancer Res. 1998;58:5453–65.
26. Wang J. Cellular roles of DNA topoisomerases: a molecular perspective. Nat Rev Mol Cell. 2002;3:430–40.
27. Heck MM, Hittelman WN, Earnshaw WC. Differential expression of DNA topoisomerases I and II during the eukaryotic cell cycle. Proc Natl Acad Sci USA. 1988;85:1086–90.

28. Suzuki A, Kato M. Chemotherapeutic agent CPT-11 induces the new expression of the apoptotic initiator to the cytoplasm. Exp Cell Res. 1996;227:154–9.
29. Rothenberg ML, Eckardt JR, Kuhn JG et al. Phase II trial of irinotecan in patients with progressive or rapidly recurrent colorectal cancer. J Clin Oncol. 1996;14:1128–35.
30. Ikuno N, Soda H, Watanabe M. Irinotecan and characteristic mucosal changes in the mouse ileum and cecum. J Natl Cancer Inst. 1995;87:1876–83.
31. Grandia D, Abigerges D, Armand JP. CPT-11 induced anticholinergic effects in cancer patients. J Clin Oncol. 1993;11:196–7.
32. Saliba F, Hagipantelli R, Misset JL et al. Pathophysiology and therapy of irinotecan-induced delayed-onset diarrhea in patients with advanced colorectal cancer: a prospective assessment. J Clin Oncol. 1998;16:2745–51.
33. Komarova EA, Chernov MV, Franks R et al. Transgenic mice with p53-responsive lacZ: p53 activity varies dramatically during normal development and determines radiation and drug sensitivity *in vivo*. EMBO J. 1997;16:1391–400.
34. Westphal CH, Rowan S, Schmaltz C, Elson A, Fisher DE, Leder P. atm and p53 cooperate in apoptosis and suppression of tumorigenesis, but not in resistance to acute radiation toxicity. Nature Genet. 1997;16:397.
35. Komarov PG, Komarova EA, Kondratov RV, Christov K, Gudkov AV. A chemical inhibitor of p53 that protects mice from side effects of cancer therapy. Science. 1999;285:1733–7.

9
Side-effects of chemotherapy on the gastrointestinal tract: symptoms, grade and classification

W. FISCHBACH

INTRODUCTION

The principles of oncological therapy comprise a curative and adjuvant intention with the goal of definite cure of the disease and relapse-free survival. Palliative therapy focuses on a better quality of life by effectively treating tumour-associated symptoms and on prolonged survival time. The therapeutic concept has to be established in any individual case before starting therapy, considering age, prognostic factors and co-morbidities. This is of the utmost importance because the therapeutic goal leads to a differentiated acceptance of chemotherapy-induced toxicities.

Oral and gastrointestinal toxicities occur as a direct result of chemotherapeutic agents and present as stomatitis, nausea and vomiting, and enteropathy. Their intensity can vary widely from minor complaints to life-threatening events. The widely used NCI (National Cancer Institute) common toxicity criteria grade chemotherapy-induced toxicities from 0 to 4. Table 1 illustrates the oral and gastrointestinal toxicities; however, there are also indirect side-effects of chemotherapy on the digestive tract. Granulocytopenia increases the risk for enteral infections, and gastrointestinal bleeding may be caused by thrombocytopenia.

NAUSEA AND VOMITING

Nausea and vomiting are not only the most frequent acute side-effects of chemotherapy; they also represent the most distressing symptoms experienced by cancer patients submitted to chemotherapy[1] (Figure 1). Despite undisputed progress during recent years, emesis remains a critical problem of chemotherapy; it may cause considerable physical and psychological consequences. Electrolyte

Table 1 NCI common toxicity criteria (for oral and gastrointestinal toxicities)

Toxicity	*Grade*				
	0	*1*	*2*	*3*	*4*
Nausea	None	Able to eat; reasonable intake	Intake decreased but can eat	No significant intake	
Vomiting	None	1 episode in 24 h	2–5 episodes in 24 h	6–10 episodes in 24 h	>10 episodes in 24 h requiring parenteral support
Stomatitis	None	Painless ulcers, erythema, or mild soreness	Painful erythema, oedema, or ulcers, but can eat	Painful erythema, oedema, or ulcers; cannot eat	Requires (par)enteral support
Diarrhoea	None	2–3 stools/day	4–6 stools/day, or nocturnal stools, or moderate cramping	7–9 stools/day, or incontinence, severe cramping	≥10 stools/day, or bloody diarrhoea, parenteral support

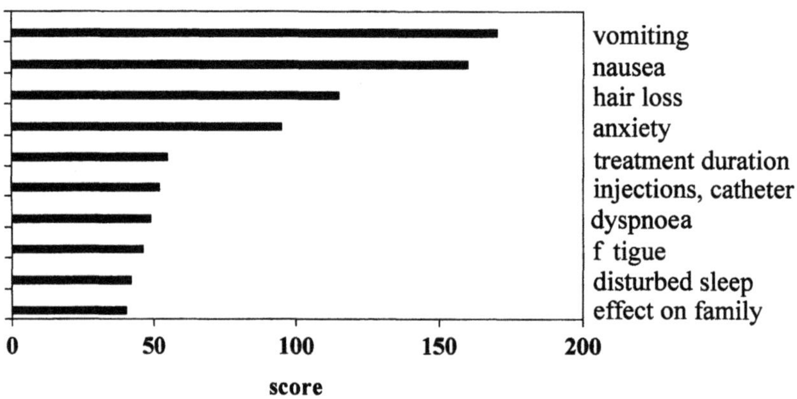

Figure 1 Strains and discomforts of chemotherapy

disturbance can be observed, and dehydration reduces renal elimination which may result in a further accumulation of the cytotoxic agent. Prolonged or remittent nausea and vomiting will lead to weight loss and increase the risk for anorexia. The patient's compliance suffers considerably from these symptoms, and cessation of therapy as a consequence of a markedly impaired quality of life may be inevitable in the individual case.

Factors that influence vomiting are

1. the cytotoxic drug and its emetic potential (Figure 2);
2. the combination of chemotherapeutic agents;
3. the dose;
4. the route of administration (oral, intravenous);
5. the schedule of administration (bolus, infusional).

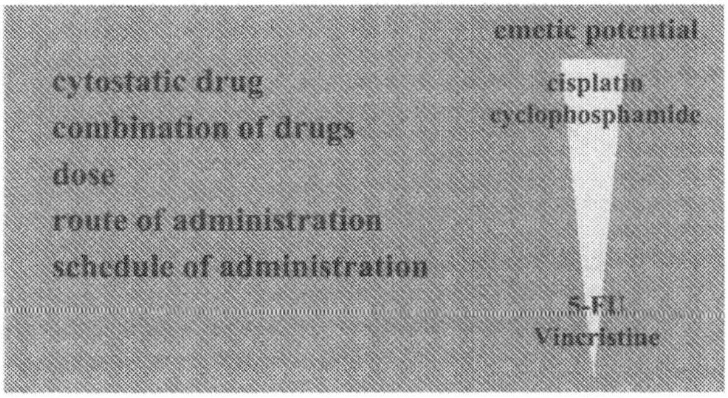

Figure 2 Factors that influence vomiting

There are four forms of emesis. Acute emesis usually begins 2–3 h after administration of the drug, reaches its maximal intensity after 5–6 h, and thereafter appears only sporadically. Prolonged (lasting up to 24 h and longer) and delayed emesis (starting 24 h after chemotherapy) are mostly associated with high doses of highly emetic cytotoxic agents. In addition to occurring after treatment, nausea and vomiting can occur before treatment. Roughly 30% of patients experience this anticipatory emesis in some series of systematic studies. Nausea and vomiting in anticipation of treatment results from an expectation anxiety based on uncontrolled emesis during prior treatment and may represent a big problem not easy to influence in a positive way.

Another cause of emesis which should be considered in the individual case is infectious oesophagitis on the basis of chemotherapy-induced immunosuppression. A time delay of symptoms after chemotherapy should focus on this differential diagnosis and cause oral inspection and endoscopic examination. Candidiasis as the most frequent cause of oesophagitis should be treated topically and systemically using antimycotics.

STOMATITIS

Stomatitis is another frequent and serious side-effect of chemotherapy; it is caused by a direct cytotoxic effect on the mucosa and usually evolves 5–6 days after administration of the agents. Common forms of indirect stomatitis are oral infection and haemorrhage; they are usually noted at the patient's nadir and thus occur 10–14 days after drug administration. There are therapy-related factors that influence the occurrence of stomatitis such as the cytotoxic drug, its dose and route of administration. A combined radiochemotherapy particularly predisposes to stomatitis. On the other hand, various individual factors characterize the patient's susceptibility: age, gender, hepatic and renal function, and the enzymal status (i.e. in the case of fluorouracil-based protocols). The oral hygienic status is of utmost importance with respect to the development of stomatitis. Some oncologists consider a dental examination necessary before starting therapy.

The clinical feature of stomatitis is characterized by oedema, erythema, erosions and ulcers. The most common sites involved are the buccal, labial, and soft palatal mucosa, along with the ventral surface of the tongue and the floor of the mouth. The major clinical problem is pain, with the inability to eat and drink requiring parenteral support in the worst cases (Table 1). It should be emphasized that continuation of chemotherapy can be considered only after complete healing of stomatitis.

CHEMOTHERAPY-ASSOCIATED ENTEROPATHY

There are two forms of chemotherapy-associated enteropathies. Neuropathy caused, for example, by vinca alkaloids may result in obstipation and paralytic ileus in the individual case. On the other hand, diarrhoea may develop on the basis of cytotoxic and inflammatory changes of the intestinal mucosa. Diarrhoea may principally follow the administration of all chemotherapeutic agents, but is most frequently found after the use of: (a) antimetabolites, such as fluorouracil and methotrexate; (b) anthracyclines, such as doxorubicin; (c) topoisomersase 1 inhibitors, such as irinotecan.

Clinically, the secretory type of diarrhoea predominates: frequent liquid stools and inefficiency of fasting procedures. The occurrence of nocturnal stools, incontinence and bloody diarrhoea characterize the grade of toxicity (Table 1) and determine the intensity of therapy. In any case of chemotherapy-associated diarrhoea, especially in the case of delayed diarrhoea, antibiotic-associated enterocolitis and infectious enterocolitis should be excluded by means of stool examination (pathogenic bacteria, *Lamblia, Clostridium difficile* toxin), serology and endoscopic–bioptic investigation.

CONCLUSION

Against the background of cure, chemotherapy-related side-effects will be accepted in a relatively generous way in the case of a curative treatment intention. Nevertheless, all symptomatic and prophylactic efforts should be made in order to avoid the risk of this therapeutic goal due to uncontrolled toxicities. In an adjuvant situation considerable malaise may not be tolerated, and therapy may be stopped for that reason, not knowing the risk of tumour relapse induced by this decision. Finally, palliative chemotherapy focuses on life quality as the decisive criterion. The possible benefit of chemotherapy on the one hand, and treatment-related complaints on the other, should be balanced in a very thorough way.

Reference

1. Coates A, Abraham S, Kaye SB et al. On the receiving end – patient perception of the side-effects of cancer chemotherapy. Eur J Cancer Clin Oncol. 1983;19:203–8.

Section IV
Adverse effects of chemotherapeutic agents – pathophysiology and therapeutic approaches

10
Central origin and psychosomatics of nausea and emesis

K. JORDAN

INTRODUCTION

Nausea and vomiting following chemotherapy are a major cause of morbidity in the oncological patient. Nausea and vomiting are two of the most distressing symptoms experienced by cancer patients undergoing chemotherapy.

The physiology and neuropharmacology of emesis was first studied in the 1950s by Borison and co-workers[1,2], forming the framework that allowed an understanding of emesis. During this period phenothiazines were introduced into practice, as in addition to their antipsychotic properties an antiemetic effect had been noted. Knowing that phenothiazines interact with dopamine receptors, and that the area postrema in the medulla oblongata is involved in emesis, gave an enhanced insight into clinical approaches.

Besides the understanding of the pathophysiology of emesis in recent decades, 20 years ago a phenomenon labelled 'anticipatory nausea and vomiting' (ANV) arose. By the fourth cycle of chemotherapy 30% of patients have developed ANV; it appears to have links to psychological, neurological and physiological systems, and cannot be explained by pharmacological factors only.

CENTRAL ORIGIN OF NAUSEA AND EMESIS

Anatomy

The central origin of chemotherapy-related emesis is mainly based on two structures in the formatio reticularis within the brainstem (Figure 1):

1. The chemoreceptor trigger zone (CTZ) is located in the area postrema at the bottom end of the fourth ventricle. The CTZ is a circumventricular organ, which basically means that this structure lacks an effective blood–brain barrier and is able to detect emetic agents in both the systemic circulation and

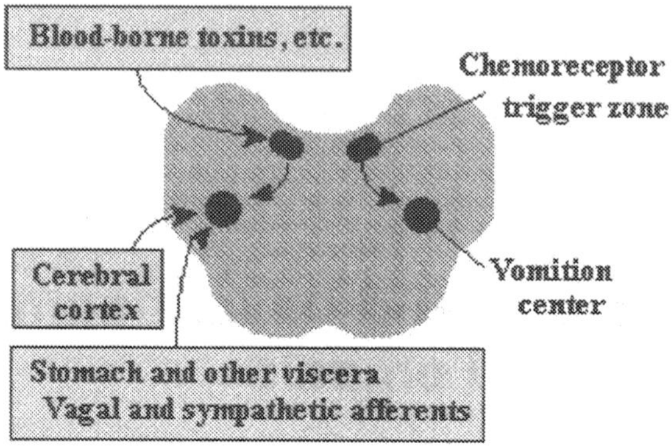

Figure 1 Chemoreceptor trigger zone and vomiting centre in the brainstem

the cerebrospinal fluid. The area postrema has afferent and efferent connections with underlying structures, the subnucleus gelatinosus and nucleus tractus solitarius, receiving vagal afferent fibres from the gastrointestinal tract[3].

2. The vomiting centre is located in the brainstem medullary structures and is a collection of effector nuclei rather than a discrete brain area. It receives major inputs from the CTZ and a vagal and sympathetic input from the gut, the cardiovascular system and a number of limbic brain nuclei.

Pathophysiology of nausea and emesis

Vomiting due to chemotherapy is the result of stimulation of a multistep reflex pathway controlled by the brain. Vomiting is triggered by afferent impulses to the vomiting centre from the CTZ, as mentioned above, the gastrointestinal tract via the vagal nerve and cerebral cortex. Vomiting occurs when efferent impulses are sent from the vomiting centre to the salivation centre, abdominal muscles, respiratory centre, and cranial nerves[4] (see Figure 2 for a schematic representation of the reflex pathways of vomiting). These pathways are mediated by neurotransmitters. The gastrointestinal tract, CTZ and vomiting centre are abundant with neurotransmitter receptors. The principal neurotransmitters involved in the emetic response are: serotonin, dopamine, and substance P (tachykinin).

Serotonin

Serotonin is the main neurotransmitter responsible for emesis after chemotherapy. The serotonin (5-HT_3) receptors are located in three sites: gastrointestinal tract, CTZ in the area postrema, and nucleus tractus solitarius of the vomiting centre. Following exposure to radiation or cytotoxic drugs, 5-HT is released from enterochromaffine cells in the small intestinal mucosa, which are adjacent to the vagal afferent neurons on which 5-HT_3 receptors are located[5] (Figure 2). The released serotonin activates vagal afferent neurons via the 5-HT_3 receptors, which leads ultimately to a severe emetic response mediated via the CTZ within the area postrema[2]. Although the vagal nerve relays information to the area

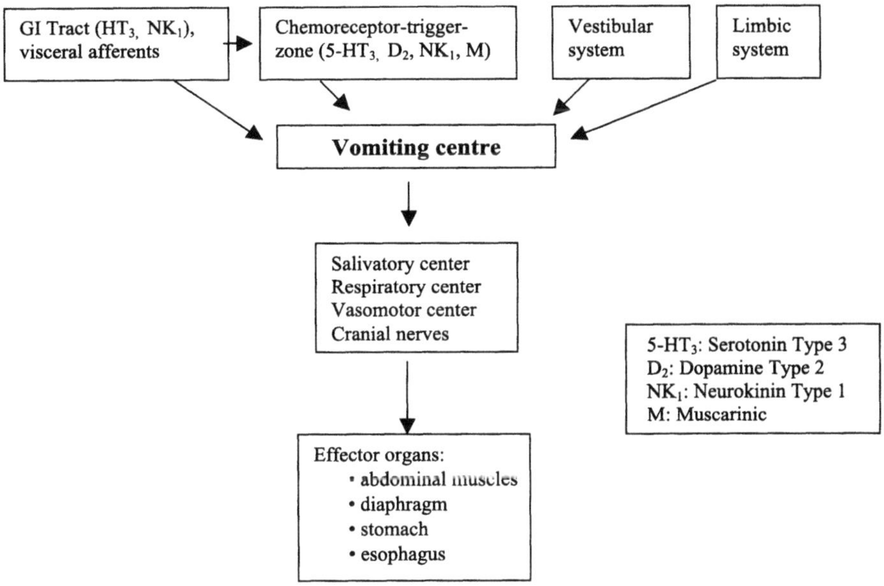

Figure 2 Reflex pathway of vomiting

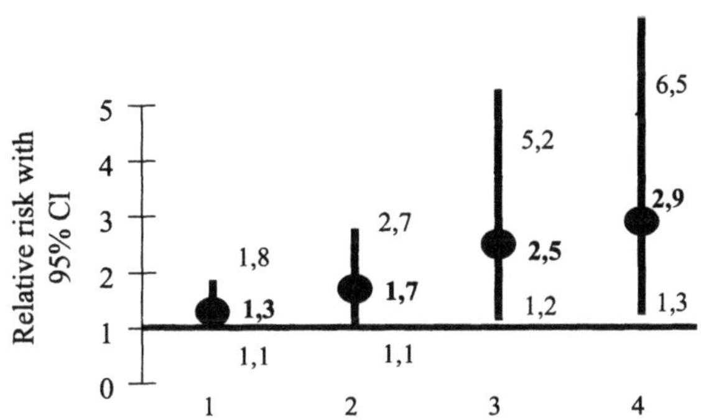

Figure 3 Potential risk for postchemotherapy nausea and vomiting (PCNV). 1, Tiredness; 2, impairment through pain in daily life; 3, gastric uneasiness; 4, impairment of daily interactions with other people

postrema, most of the sensory information from the vagal nerve is relayed to the tractus solitarius of the vomiting centre.

Another pathway is direct stimulation of the CTZ with cytotoxic agents. This is due to the fact that the CTZ as a circumventricular organ lies outside the blood–brain barrier; therefore it can detect chemical stimuli from both the blood and the cerebrospinal fluid. Subsequently, the CTZ transmits a signal to the vomiting centre.

Dopamine

Dopamine interacts with dopamine D_1 and D_2 receptors, whereas the dopamine D_2 receptor, located in the CTZ, is responsible for chemotherapy-induced emesis. In early antiemetic trials in the 1960s attention was mostly paid to agents that block dopamine receptors[6]. Today it is recognized that the antiemetic effect of high-dose metoclopramide is probably due to 5-HT_3 receptor antagonism, whereas adverse events and the effect of low doses are caused by antagonism of the dopamine D_2 receptor[7].

Substance P

Recent research has focused on the potential role of neuropeptides in the vomiting reflexes. Substance P, an 11-amino-acid neuropeptide, has been localized within the area postrema, nucleus tractus solitarius, and gastrointestinal tract, and is released in response to noxious stimuli. Substance P exerts its effects by binding to the neurokinin-1 (NK-1) receptor. The development of non-peptide NK-1 antagonists, which cross the blood–brain barrier, has offered the opportunity to target antiemetics acting upon the substance P pathway. These antagonists are still being evaluated as antiemetics for the prophylaxis of chemotherapy-induced acute and especially delayed emesis. The NK_1 antagonists are able to antagonize a much broader spectrum of emetic stimuli than the 5-HT_3 receptor antagonists. It can block the emetic effect of apomorphine, morphine, nicotine, copper sulphate, ipecac, radiation, cylophosphamide, cisplatin, motion and anaesthesia in the ferret[8].

Other neuroreceptors

Other neuroreceptors involved in the emetic response, including corticosteroids, acetylcholine and histamine receptors, are located in the vomiting and vestibular centres of the brain. The mechanism of action of corticosteroids still remains unclear. Corticosteroids might modify the capillary permeability of the chemoreceptor trigger zone[9]. The anti-inflammatory properties of corticosteroids may act as an antiemetic by preventing the release of serotonin in the gut or preventing the activation of 5-HT_3 receptors in the gastrointestinal tract[10]. They may also have a role in endorphin release[11].

Antihistamines and anticholinergics have failed to prove antiemetic activity due to chemotherapy. They are used to prevent the extrapyramidal side-effects that can occur in response to dopamine D_2 receptor antagonists. Both play a role in controlling nausea and vomiting in patients susceptible to motion sickness.

PSYCHOSOMATIC

Nausea and vomiting after chemotherapy cannot be explained only by receptor-associated pathways. Among patients receiving the same chemotherapy at equivalent doses, considerably different levels of post-treatment nausea and vomiting have been reported. Several risk factors such as age, sex, previous history of motion sickness, and alcohol consumption have been identified. To obtain a more exact understanding of these individual differences we must focus on the concept of anticipatory nausea and vomiting, as well as the influence of other psychological factors.

Anticipatory nausea and vomiting

The phenomenon of anticipatory nausea and vomiting (ANV) has mainly been investigated by Morrow and his colleagues[12,13]. Approximately 15 years ago it was noted that some patients showed nausea and emesis prior to a second or subsequent cycle of chemotherapy, and once patients develop ANV it cannot be controlled by pharmacological means. The prevalence of anticipatory nausea and vomiting by the fourth cycle of chemotherapy has been reported in 30% of patients.

Aetiology

Several characteristics of ANV suggested that its mechanisms might fit within a learning model, and it was later confirmed that the development of ANV involves elements of classical conditioning[14]. Classical conditioning is also known as Pavlovian conditioning, named after the Russian scientist Pavlov. During the years 1891 and 1900 Pavlov looked at the digestive process in dogs, especially the interaction between salivation and the action of the stomach. He realized that they were closely linked by reflexes in the autonomic nervous system. Without salivation the stomach did not get the message to start digesting. Pavlov saw that he could initiate this salivation without the stimulus of food. He rang a bell whenever he gave the dog the experimental food. Eventually he stopped giving the dogs food, but rang the bell regardless; and the dogs would begin to salivate even though there was no food present. Pavlov called this response a conditioned reflex. How is this transferable to chemotherapy and emesis?

Potential conditioned stimuli, such as the sight of the nurse, or other sights are present while the chemotherapy (unconditioned stimulus) that produces the unconditioned response – nausea and vomiting – is given. Over several chemotherapy cycles the conditioned response stimuli (sights, sounds) can be learned; they then produce what is now called the conditioned response of ANV[15].

The onset of ANV increases almost linearly with the number of chemotherapy cycles administered, and is related to both the frequency and the severity of post-treatment nausea and vomiting[16].

Treatment of ANV

In general it can be stated that antiemetics do not control ANV once it has developed. Furthermore some studies showed a paradox increase of symptoms after giving antiemetics, so some investigators saw the antiemetics themselves as a conditioned stimulus[17]. Some authors suggested a preventive intervention with benzodiazepines.

If anticipatory emesis occurs, behavioural therapy with systematic desensitization (SD) is recommended[12,18]. A key element of SD is to construct a hierarchy of occasions related to the original stimulus which elict the maladaptive response in each patient. This hierarchy might include events related to the receipt of chemotherapy, such as driving to the clinic, entering the chemotherapy room, and seeing the clinic nurse. Following this, the patient is trained to associate an alternative response (e.g. deep muscle relaxation) with these events[19].

Other psychological factors

Although the reasons for failure to achieve complete control may be explained by a better understanding of the underlying physiological and pharmacological mechanisms, an association between emesis and psychosocial factors should also be considered. Only a few studies within recent years have examined the possible association between patients' health-related quality of life (HQoL) characteristics and postchemotherapy nausea and vomiting (PCNV). Osoba et al. discovered that prechemotherapy HQoL scores in several domains were significantly different in patients who experienced PCNV as compared with patients who had no PCNV[20]. Specifically, this study showed that patients with pre-existing pain; insomnia; impaired emotional, cognitive and social function are at a higher risk of developing postchemotherapy nausea and vomiting.

In a small study with 43 patients receiving moderately or highly emetogenic chemotherapy we examined QoL factors with a QoL questionnaire, similar to the QLQ-30, prior to chemotherapy. Patients with tiredness, those impaired by pain in their daily life, with gastric uneasiness and with impairment of daily interactions with other people had a significantly higher relative risk of developing nausea and vomiting after chemotherapy (Figure 3)[21].

References

1. Borison HL, Brand ED, Orkand RK. Emetic action of nitrogen mustard (mechlorethamine hydrochloride) in dogs and cats. Am J Physiol. 1958;192:410–16.
2. Borison HL, Wang S. Physiology and pharmacology of vomiting. Pharmacol Rev. 1953;5:193–230.
3. Leslie RA. Comparative aspects of the area postrema: fine structural considerations help determine its function. Cell Mol Neurobiol. 1986;6:95–120.
4. Craig JB, Powell BL. The management of nausea and vomiting in clinical oncology. Am J Med Sci. 1987;293:43–4.
5. Andrews PLR. The pharmacologic profile of granisetron (Kytril). Semin Oncol. 1994;21:3–9.
6. Gralla RJ. The evolution of antiemetic treatment. In: Dicato AM, editor. Medical Management of Cancer Treatment Induced Emesis. London: Dunitz, 1998:1–7.
7. Herrstedt J. Dopamine antagonists and other agents. In: Extended abstract book. Consensus conference on antiemetic therapy. Perugia, 1997:52–9.
8. Hesketh PJ. Potential role of the NK1 receptor antagonists in chemotherapy-induced nausea and vomiting. Support Care Cancer. 2001;9:350–4.
9. Livera P, Trojano M, Simone IL. Acute changes in blood CSF barrier permselectivity to serum proteins after intrathecal methotrexate and CNS irradiation. J Neurol. 1985;231:336–9.
10. Fredrikson M, Hursti T, Furst CJ. Nausea in cancer chemotherapy is inversely related to urinary cortisol excretion. Br J Cancer. 1992;65:779–80.
11. Harris AL. Cytotoxic-therapy induced vomiting is mediated via enkephalin pathways. Lancet. 1982;1:714.
12. Morrow GR, Asbury R, Hammon S. Comparing the effectiveness of behavioral treatment for chemotherapy-induced nausea and vomiting when administered by oncologists, oncology nurses, and clinical psychologists. Health Psychol. 1992;11:250–6.

13. Morrow GR, Roscoe JA. Anticipatory nausea and vomiting: models, mechanisms and management. In: Dicato AM, editor. Medical Management of Cancer Treatment Induced Emesis. London: Dunitz, 1998:149–66.
14. Carey MP, Burish TG. Etiology and treatment of psychological side effects associated with cancer chemotherapy: a critical review and discussion. Psychol Bull. 1988;104:307–25.
15. Morrow GR, Rosenthal SN. Models, mechanisms and management of anticipatory nausea and emesis. Oncology. 1996;53:4–7.
16. Tomoyasu N, Bovbjerg DH, Jacobsen PB. Conditioned reactions to cancer chemotherapy: percent reinforcement predicts anticipatory nausea. Physiol Behav. 1996;2:273–6.
17. Morrow GR, Arsenau JC, Asbury RF, Bennett JM, Boros L. Anticipatory nausea and vomiting with chemotherapy. N Engl J Med. 1982;306:431–2.
18. Burish TG, Carey MP, Krozely MG. Conditioned side effects induced by cancer chemotherapy: prevention through behavioral treatment. J Consult Clin Psychol. 1987;55:42–8.
19. Morrow GR, Dobkin PL. Anticipatory nausea and vomiting in cancer patients undergoing chemotherapy treatment: prevalence, etiology, and behavioral interventions. Clin Psych Rev. 1988;8:517–56.
20. Osoba D, Zee B, Pater J, Warr D, Latreille J, Kaizer L. Determinants of postchemotherapy nausea and vomiting in patients with cancer. J Clin Oncol. 1997;15:116–23.
21. Jordan K. Analyse der Granisetron- und Dexamethasongabe als Suspensionslösung in der supportiven Tumortherapie unter Berücksichtigung der Lebensqualität als Einflußfaktor auf Übelkeit und Erbrechen. Dissertation, 2001.

11
Cancer anorexia–cachexia syndrome – evidence in pathophysiology and management

A. RÜHL

INTRODUCTION

The majority of patients with advanced cancer lose weight and exhibit to some extent the features of cachexia. The prevalence of cachexia exceeds 70% for certain types of cancer, and weight loss has been shown to be more common in patients with lung and gastrointestinal cancer and less common in patients with haematological malignancies and breast cancer[1]. At the time of diagnosis 80% of patients with upper gastrointestinal cancer and 60% of patients with lung cancer have already experienced substantial weight loss[2]. Weight loss influences the tolerability of and response to chemotherapy[1,3] and the duration of survival[4,5]; indeed, weight loss appears to be a powerful independent prognostic factor[1], and in more than 20% of cancer patients cachexia is the main cause of death[2,6].

In general, cancer patients lose weight due to a reduction in food intake, an increase in energy expenditure or a combination of the two. Energy intake has been shown to be substantially reduced among weight-losing cancer patients[7]. Reduction in nutritional intake may be due to gastrointestinal dysfunctioning related to physical obstruction including malignant bowel obstruction or malabsorption, or it can be due to symptoms related to either the disease or the treatment, such as nausea, vomiting, constipation, diarrhoea, taste changes, depression or pain. Cancer-associated hypercalcaemia is a fairly common medical emergency and leads to nausea, vomiting and loss of appetite. However, even if all of these clinical problems are appropriately controlled, cancer patients may still report early satiety and poor appetite.

Although the range of body weight is wide, the range of individual weight fluctuations over time has been shown to be rather narrow, with 95% confidence intervals for change in body weight in healthy adults of approximately ±5% within a 6-month period[8]. This reflects a tight control of body weight via adaptation of energy intake and/or energy expenditure depending on the actual nutritional status, with weight loss being a potent stimulus to food intake. The persistence of anorexia in cancer patients therefore implies a failure of this adaptive feeding response which may be associated with increased activity of proinflammatory cytokines, such as tumour necrosis factor α (TNF-α), interleukin-1β (IL-1β), interleukin-6 (IL-6) and interferon-γ (IFN-γ) or central corticotropin-releasing factor (CRF) which is a potent anorexigenic signal[9–13].

PATHOGENESIS OF THE CANCER ANOREXIA–CACHEXIA SYNDROME

Leptin, the product of the obese (*ob*) gene[14], is a peptide hormone that is secreted by adipocytes and which plays a central role in the adaptive feeding response to starvation: starvation-related weight loss causes leptin levels to fall, which in turn increases the activity of hypothalamic orexigenic signals that stimulate feeding and suppress energy expenditure (see below), and decrease the activity of anorexigenic signals that suppress appetite and increase energy expenditure[15,16]. In cancer patients the proinflammatory cytokines IL-1β, TNF-α, LIF and CNTF have been shown to interfere with this adaptive decrease in leptin levels, thus disrupting a crucial compensatory mechanism in the face of both decreased food intake and body weight[7,15].

Leptin has been shown to influence food intake and energy expenditure via neuropeptidergic effector molecules in the hypothalamus[15,16]. Complex interactions between the central nervous, endocrine, and immune systems affect the leptin loop and have a potential role in cancer-related anorexia and cachexia; specifically, it has been demonstrated that leptin is a potent suppressor of neuropeptide Y (NPY) synthesis[17]. Hypothalamic NPY is the most potent feeding-stimulatory peptide and belongs to an interconnected orexigenic network in the hypothalamus that includes galanin, opioid peptides, melanin-concentrating hormone (MCH), orexin, and agouti-related peptide (AGRP)[15,16]. In addition to leptin, the endogenous hypercytokinaemia associated with advanced cancer prevents fasting-induced up-regulation of NPY gene expression in the hypothalamus[18], and several lines of evidence suggest that NPY may be one of the key neural pathways disrupted in the cytokine-related anorexia–cachexia syndrome[15,16,18], even though there are other studies implicating additional orexigenic and/or anorexigenic signals in anorexia and body weight loss.

The orexigenic and anorexigenic neuropeptides decrease and increase sympathetic nervous activity, respectively, which regulates energy expenditure by activating thermogenesis in brown adipose tissue and possibly in other sites such as white adipose tissue and muscle[15].

Another major appetite-modulating neurotransmitter is serotonin (5-HT). Plentiful serotonergic nerve fibres and terminals lie close to or terminate on NPY-containing neurons in the hypothalamus[19]. Serotonin is a potent anorectic agent which can cause carbohydrate aversion, reduce feeding and increase energy expenditure[19]. Serotonin may play a role in the development of cancer anorexia due to increased levels of plasma and brain tryptophan, the precursor amino acid for serotonin, and increased levels of IL-1β may further increase serotonergic activity[15].

Indeed, it has been suggested that serotonergic neurotransmitter systems represent a converging final pathway of orexigenic and anorexigenic stimuli[15,19]. However, the precise mechanisms of these neuroimmune interactions have yet to be elucidated.

EVIDENCE-BASED MANAGEMENT OF THE CANCER ANOREXIA–CACHEXIA SYNDROME

Nutritional approach

The best way to treat cancer cachexia is to cure the cancer, but unfortunately this is not feasible in most patients with advanced solid tumours. As energy intake is considerably reduced in weight-losing cancer patients[7], it seems apparent that the provision of nutritional support to the malnourished patient with cancer is essential and would be beneficial – however, evidence for this is lacking.

It was hoped that enteral or parenteral nutritional support would circumvent cancer anorexia and ameliorate malnutrition. However, the inability of hypercaloric feeding to increase body weight has been repeatedly shown – regardless of whether artificial nutrition was provided via the enteral or parenteral route – and numerous prospective randomized controlled trials have been disappointing[20–33]. Artificial nutrition has neither been able to improve survival nor to decrease chemotherapy-induced toxicity. Rather, specifically in parenteral nutrition, there was an increase in infectious and mechanical complications[24–33].

However, there may be a small but important subset of patients with weight loss primarily because the gastrointestinal tract is obstructed, given that their cancer is amenable to therapy. In these patients progressive nutritional deprivation is the main mechanism of cachexia, hence in these patients parenteral or enteral nutrition will improve survival[34].

Pharmacological approach

Drugs with proven efficacy

Glucocorticoids

Glucocorticoids are widely used in the palliative setting for symptoms associated with cancer[35–38]. There have been a number of prospective, randomized, placebo-controlled trials proving symptomatic efficacy of different types of corticosteroids[35–38]. In general, corticosteroids have been shown to have a limited effect of up to 4 weeks on symptoms such as appetite, food intake, sensation of well-being, and performance status. Furthermore, all studies have failed to show any beneficial effect on body weight. Prolonged treatment may lead to weakness, delirium, osteoporosis, and immunosuppression, all of which may already be present in advanced cancer patients. Owing to their short-lasting but significant benefits, corticosteroids can be used in patients with short expected survival in whom weight gain is not a likely outcome.

The mechanism of action of glucocorticoids on appetite includes the inhibition of proinflammatory cytokines such as TNF-α and IL-1β which decrease energy intake directly or via other anorexigenic mediators, such as leptin, CRF, and serotonin (see above)[15]. Glucocorticosteroids can augment NPY levels in the hypothalamus, which appear to be responsible, at least in part, for the increased appetite and food intake (see above)[15].

Progestational drugs
Megestrol acetate (MA) and medroxyprogesterone acetate (MPA) are synthetic, orally active derivatives of the naturally occurring hormone progesterone. In several clinical trials these compounds have been found to improve appetite, caloric intake, and nutritional status[37–39]. There is, at present, considerable evidence for the effect of synthetic progestins on appetite and body weight, which has been confirmed in a recent meta-analysis[40]. Furthermore, it is recognized that these compounds may enhance appetite and cause body weight gain via stimulation of NPY[37,41]. Finally, there are reports to suggest that the positive effects of progestational drugs on appetite and body weight in cancer cachexia and anorexia are mediated by down-regulation of proinflammatory cytokines[11].

MA has demonstrated a dose-related benefit from dosages ranging from 160 mg to 1600 mg with an optimal dosage of 800 mg daily[37,40]. It is recommended that a patient be started on the lowest dosage (160 mg/day) and the dose be titrated upwards according to the clinical response. Reported side-effects of progestational drugs include thromboembolic complications, fluid retention with the development of peripheral oedema, hyperglycaemia, arterial hypertension, breakthrough uterine bleeding, and adrenal suppression with adrenal insufficiency developing if the compounds are abruptly discontinued[37,40].

Prokinetic agents
Many patients with advanced cancer have symptoms of delayed gastric emptying and gastric retention of food. In these circumstances the prokinetic agent metoclopramide (MCP) may relieve anorexia and early satiety with minimal side-effects[6,37]. The role of other prokinetic agents needs to be examined in randomized trials in cancer patients.

Drugs without proven efficacy

Pentoxifylline
Pentoxifylline, a methylxanthine derivative, is a phosphodiesterase inhibitor that has been shown to inhibit TNF-α synthesis by decreasing gene transcription. In a randomized, double-blind and placebo-controlled trial in patients with cancer cachexia, pentoxifylline failed to demonstrate any benefit in terms of appetite or nutritional measures compared to placebo[42]. Most likely this finding reflects that TNF-suppression alone is not sufficient to reverse the activation of the various mediator pathways involved in the cancer anorexia–cachexia syndrome. However, it is also conceivable that the TNF-antagonism exerted by pentoxifylline does not sufficiently block this powerful proinflammatory cytokine to revert its effects in CACS.

Dronabinol
After numerous anecdotal reports and small studies suggesting appetite-stimulating efficacy for cannabinoids, and one promising phase II trial of delta-9-tetrahydrocannabinol (THC; dronabinol)[43], a large double-blind randomized NCCTG study

was undertaken to compare the effects of dronabinol alone or in combination with megestrol acetate (MA) with MA alone[44]. In this study MA clearly provided superior palliation of anorexia in advanced cancer patients than dronabinol alone, and combination therapy did not confer additional benefit[44].

Anabolic steroids

Anabolic steroids increase muscle mass in non-cancer patients and have hence been proposed for the treatment of cancer cachexia. However, in a large, randomized, controlled trial comparing megestrol acetate versus dexamethasone versus fluoxymesterone for the treatment of the cancer anorexia–cachexia syndrome, fluoxymesterone was clearly inferior[45].

Emerging drugs

Thalidomide

Thalidomide has been found to successfully inhibit TNF-α in animals and humans with cancer, AIDS, and other diseases. In these conditions thalidomide treatment has been shown to result in a significant improvement in well-being as well as appetite, with reduction in nausea[37,46]. These results, together with the recent finding that thalidomide is able to inhibit cancer growth through an inhibition of neo-angiogenesis, suggests a unique role of this compound both as an anticachectic and antineoplastic agent.

Melatonin

Melatonin is a pineal hormone that is able to decrease the level of circulating TNF-α in patients with advanced cancer. In a recent controlled trial of 100 patients with metastatic solid tumours, loss of more than 10% body weight was less common among patients treated with melatonin than among patients in the placebo group[37].

Non-pharmacological approach

Physical activity in patients with cancer

As shown in a systematic review of exercise intervention studies in patients with advanced cancer, physical exercise can significantly improve quality of life, functional capacity, muscle strength, and body composition in this patient group[47]. As physical activity has also been reported to be beneficial for outcome parameters such as fatigue, anxiety and depression in advanced cancer, physical exercise appears worthwhile to be examined in large randomized trials in cancer patients.

CONCLUSIONS

Our knowledge of the complex biology of the cancer anorexia–cachexia syndrome is growing. In recent years the cancer anorexia–cachexia syndrome has been understood to be the result of major metabolic abnormalities due to a combination of host cytokine release and tumour by-products, rather than as a simple increase in energy consumption by the tumour and starvation by the patient.

However, the precise mechanisms of the underlying neuroimmune and metabolic interactions have yet to be elucidated.

At present it is evident that there will be no single therapeutic solution for this condition, but perhaps combined multimodal therapy based on our understanding of the underlying biology may provide significant progress in the future. Conceivable multimodal approaches could combine nutritional support with pharmacological modulation of metabolism and/or inflammation and physical exercise[10].

References

1. DeWys WD, Begg C, Lavin PT et al. Prognostic effect of weight loss prior to chemotherapy in cancer patients. Am J Med. 1980;69:491–7.
2. Bruera E. Anorexia, cachexia and nutrition. Br Med J. 1997;315:1219–22.
3. Copeland EM III, Daly JM, Dudrick SJ. Nutrition as an adjuvant to cancer treatment in the adult. Cancer Res. 1977;37:2451–6.
4. Byar D, Kenis Y, Van Andel JG et al. Results of a E.O.R.T.C. randomized trial of cyclophosphamide and radiotherapy in inoperable lung cancer: Prognostic factors and treatment results. Eur J Cancer. 1978;14:919–30.
5. Lanzotti VJ, Thomas DR, Boyle LE, Smith TL, Gelman EA, Samuels ML. Survival with inoperable lung cancer – integration of prognostic variables based on simple clinical criteria. Cancer. 1977;39:303–13.
6. Davis MP, Dickerson D. Cachexia and anorexia: cancer's covert killer. Support Care Cancer. 2000;8:180–7.
7. Wigmore SJ, Plester CE, Ross JA et al. Contribution of anorexia and hypermetabolism to weight loss in anicteric patients with pancreatic cancer. Br J Surg. 1997;84:196–7.
8. Kotler DP. Cachexia. Ann Intern Med. 2000;133:622–34.
9. Moldawer LL, Rogy MA, Lowry SF. The role of cytokines in cancer cachexia. J Parent Ent Nutr. 1992;16:43–9.
10. Moldawer LL, Copeland EM 3rd. Proinflammatory cytokines, nutritional support, and the cachexia syndrome: interactions and therapeutic options. Cancer. 1997;79:1828–39.
11. Mantovani G, Maccio A, Lai P et al. Cytokine activity in cancer-related anorexia/cachexia: role of megestrol acetate and medroxyprogesterone acetate. Semin Oncol. 1998;25:45–52.
12. Tache Y, Garrick T, Raybould H. Central nervous system action of peptides to influence gastrointestinal motor function. Gastroenterology. 1990;98:517–28.
13. Fujimiya M, Inui A. Peptidergic regulation of gastrointestinal motility in rodents. Peptides. 2000;21:1565–82.
14. Zhang Y, Proenca R, Maffei M, Barone M, Leopold L, Friedman JM. Positional cloning of the mouse obese gene and its human homologue. Nature. 1994;372:425–32.
15. Inui A. Cancer anorexia–cachexia syndrome: are neuropeptides the key? Cancer Res. 1999;59:4493–501.
16. Woods SC, Seeley RJ, Porte D Jr et al. Signals that regulate food intake and energy homeostasis. Science. 1998;280:1378–83.
17. Stephens TW, Basinski M, Bristow PK et al. The role of neuropeptide Y in the antiobesity action of the *obese* gene product. Nature. 1995;377:530–2.
18. Sonti G, Ilyin SE, Plata-Salaman CR. Anorexia induced by cytokine interactions at pathophysiological concentrations. Am J Physiol. 1996;270:1349–402.
19. Dryden S, Frankish HM, Wang Q, Pickavance L, Williams G. The serotonergic agent fluoxetine reduces neuropeptide Y levels and neuropeptide Y secretion in the hypothalamus of lean and obese rats. Neuroscience. 1996;72:557–66.
20. Elkort RJ, Baker FL, Vitale JJ et al. Long-term nutritional support as an adjunct to chemotherapy for breast cancer. J Parent Ent Nutr. 1981;5:385.
21. Evans WK, Nixon DW, Dlay JM et al. A randomized study of oral nutritional support versus *ad lib* nutritional intake during chemotherapy for advanced colorectal and non-small cell lung cancer. J Clin Oncol. 1987;5:113.

22. Tandon SP, Gupta SC, Sinha SN et al. Nutritional support as an adjunct therapy of advanced cancer patients. Indian J Med Res. 1984;80:180.
23. Bounous G, Gentile JM, Hugon J. Elemental diet in the management of the intestinal lesion produced by 5-fluorouracil in man. Can J Surg. 1971;14:312.
24. Nixon DW, Moffitt S, Lawson DH et al. Total parenteral nutrition as an adjunct to chemotherapy of metastatic colorectal cancer. Cancer Treat Rep. 1981;65(Suppl. 5):121.
25. Nixon DW, Heymsfield SB, Lawson DH et al. Effect of total parenteral nutrition on survival in advanced colon cancer. Cancer Detect Prev. 1981;4:421.
26. Samuels ML, Selig DE, Ogden S et al. IV hyperalimentation and chemotherapy for stage II testicular cancer: a randomized study. Cancer Treat Rep. 1981;65:615.
27. Shamberger RC, Brennan MF, Goodgame JT et al. A prospective, randomized study of adjuvant parenteral nutrition in the treatment of sarcoma: results of metabolic and survival studies. Surgery. 1984;96:1.
28. Shamberger RC, Pizzo PA, Goodgame JT et al. The effect of total parenteral nutrition on chemotherapy-induced myelosuppression. Am J Med. 1983;74:40.
29. Valdivieso M, Frankmann C, Murphy WK et al. Long-term effects of intravenous hyperalimentation administered during intensive chemotherapy for small cell bronchogenic carcinoma. Cancer. 1987;59:362.
30. Valdivieso M, Bodey GP, Benjamin RS et al. Role of intravenous hyperalimentation as an adjunct to intensive chemotherapy for small cell bronchogenic carcinoma. Cancer Treat Rep. 1981;65(Suppl. 5):145.
31. Clamon GH, Feld R, Evans WK et al. Effect of adjuvant central IV hyperalimentation on the survival and response to treatment of patients with small cell lung cancer: a randomized trial. Cancer Treat Rep. 1985;69:167.
32. Issell BF, Valdivieso MD, Zaren HA et al. Protection against chemotherapy toxicity by IV hyperalimentation. Cancer Treat Rep. 1978;62:1139.
33. Jordán WM, Valdivieso M, Frankmann C et al. Treatment of advanced adenocarcinoma of the lung with ftorafur, doxorubicin, cyclophosphamide, and cisplatin (FACP) and intensive IV hyperalimentation. Cancer Treat Rep. 1981;65:197.
34. Nelson KA. The cancer anorexia–cachexia syndrome. Semin Oncol. 2000;27:64–8.
35. Moertel CG, Schutt AJ, Reitemeier RJ et al. Corticosteroid therapy of preterminal gastrointestinal cancer. Cancer. 1974;33:1607–9.
36. Bruera E, Roca E, Cedaro L et al. Action of oral methylprednisolone in terminal cancer patients: a prospective randomized double-blind study. Cancer Treat Rep. 1985;69:751–4.
37. Gagnon B, Bruera E. A review of the drug treatment of cachexia associated with cancer. Drugs. 1998;55:675–88.
38. Mantovani G, Maccio A, Massa E et al. Managing cancer-related anorexia/cachexia. Drugs. 2001;61:499–514.
39. Loprinzi CL, Michalak JC, Schaid DJ et al. Phase III evaluation of four doses of megestrol acetate as therapy for patients with cancer anorexia and/or cachexia. J Clin Oncol. 1993;11:762–7.
40. Maltoni M, Nanni O, Scarpi E et al. High-dose progestins for the treatment of cancer anorexia–cachexia syndrome: a systematic review of randomised clinical trials. Ann Oncol. 2001;12:289–300.
41. McCarthy HD, Crowder RE, Dryden S, Williams G. Megestrol acetate stimulates food and water intake in the rat: effects on regional hypothalamic neuropeptide Y concentrations. Eur J Pharmacol. 1994;265:99–102.
42. Goldberg RM, Loprinzi CI, Maillard JA et al. Pentoxifylline for treatment of cancer anorexia and cachexia? A randomized, double-blind, placebo-controlled trial. J Clin Oncol. 1995;13: 2856–9.
43. Nelson K, Walsh D, Deeter P et al. A phase II study of delta-9-tetrahydrocannabinol for appetite stimulation in cancer-associated anorexia. J Palliat Care. 1994;10:14–18.
44. Jatoi A, Windschitl HE, Loprinzi CL et al. Dronabinol versus megestrol acetate versus combination therapy for cancer-associated anorexia: a North Central Cancer Treatment Group study. J Clin Oncol. 2002;20:567–73.
45. Loprinzi CL, Kugler JW, Sloan JA et al. Randomized comparison of megestrol acetate versus dexamethasone versus fluoxymesterone for the treatment of cancer anorexia/cachexia. J Clin Oncol. 1999;17:3299–306.

46. Tramontana JM, Utaipat U, Molloy A et al. Thalidomide treatment reduces tumor necrosis factor alpha production and enhances weight gain in patients with pulmonary tuberculosis. Mol Med. 1995;1:384–97.
47. Courneya KS, Friedenreich CM. Physical exercise and quality of life following cancer diagnosis: a literature review. Ann Behav Med. 1999;21:171–9.

12
Mucositis

J. T. HARTMANN and H.-P. LIPP

INTRODUCTION

Mucositis is often a painful, debilitating, dose-limiting side-effect of cancer chemotherapy. Approximately 40% (range 20–75%) of patients undergoing cancer chemotherapy experience acute or chronic oral complications. With the evaluability of dose-intensive chemotherapy and interdisciplinary treatment concepts the importance of oral mucositis as a significant side-effect has increased. Mucositis is a common term for the oral symptoms the oncology patient develops during the course of chemotherapy, but mucositis is not simply the result of mucosal ulcerations from chemotherapy. Oral pain has multiple aetiologies arising from dental apparatus, soft tissues or bones. The oral mucosa can be directly damaged by cytoreductive therapies. This disruption in mucosal barrier function in a myelosuppressed cancer patient can lead to systemic infections[1]. Disturbances in salivary gland function can result in increased levels of pathogens colonizing the oral tissues, and may contribute to the risk of systemic complications. Despite the biological complexity of oral toxicity of chemotherapy, appropriate oral interventions before myelosuppressive cancer treatment, combined with comprehensive care of the oral cavity during or after that treatment, result in reduced morbidity and mortality. This is of increasing importance because oral ulcerative mucositis is a significant and common risk factor for bacteraemia, which results in longer hospital stay and increased costs, especially in patients who have received bone marrow transplantation[2–4].

PATHOPHYSIOLOGY

The pathogenesis of mucositis is complex[5]. Stomatotoxic chemotherapy (and/or radiation) initiates a parallel and sequential series of events that results in injury. The generation of oxygen-free radicals and DNA damage are primary events in the process, triggering a variety of signal pathways that result in downstream events. Electron microscopic evidence suggests that early changes occur in both the endothelium of submucosal blood vessels and connective tissue, although mucositis is generally considered to be an epithelial process. It seems probable that damage to connective tissue leads to a disruption of fibronectin. This can result in stimulation of proinflammatory cytokines (e.g. tumour necrosis factor alpha (TNF-α)) and production of potentially destructive metalloproteinases.

CLINICAL PRESENTATION OF MUCOSITIS

Patients suffering from mucositis often describe a burning sensation in the mouth within 3–10 days after the initiation of chemotherapy. This frequently precedes objective signs and should alert the clinician to the problem. Any of the mucosal surfaces may then develop erythema and progress to erosion and ulceration over the next 3–5 days. Intensive pain, inability to handle secretions and severe reduction in oral intake may result. The damage is usually reversible, with self-healing occurring over the next 1–2 weeks following completion of therapy (see Figure 1).

AGENTS CAUSING MUCOSITIS

A variety of chemotherapeutic agents affect rapidly proliferating cells and may produce stomatitis, cheilosis, glossitis, oesophagitis, and oral ulceration, all of which may decrease dietary intake. The frequency and severity of mucositis depends on the particular antineoplastic drug and its dose, schedule and regimen

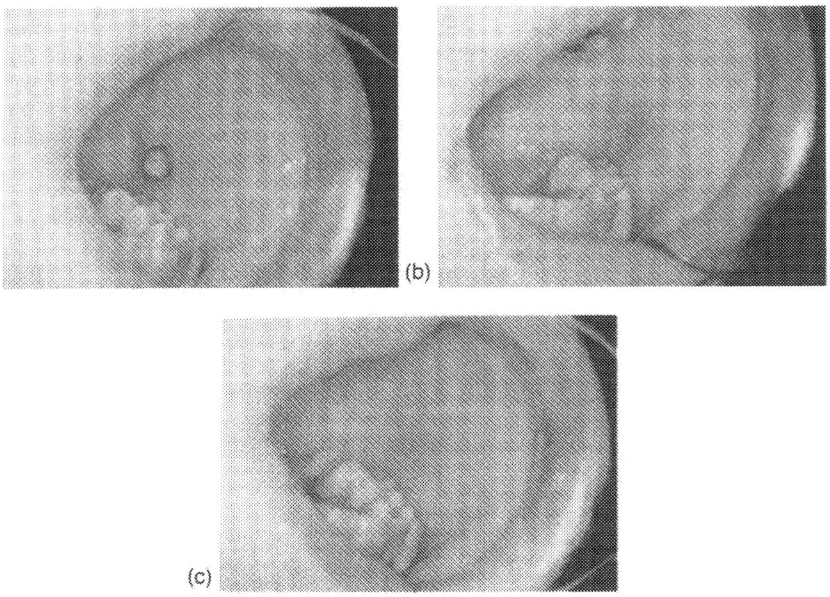

(a) (b) (c)

Figure 1 Oral mucositis in a cancer patient receiving chemotherapy: (**a**) day 1 after nadir of granulocytes, (**b**) day 8: beginning of self-healing of the ulcus, (**c**) day 15: complete healing (i.e. given alone or in combination with other cytotoxic agents or radiation therapy). Mucositis is commonly caused by methotrexate, the antibiotic antitumour agents (particularly adriamycin and actinomycin D), 5-fluorouracil (5-FU), especially when given as short injection (bolus), and the vinca alkaloids (see Table 1).

The toxicity of methotrexate to the gastrointestinal epithelium and other normal tissues depends on the duration of exposure to cytotoxic concentrations of the drug rather than to the peak levels achieved[6]. Disappearance of methotrexate from plasma following an intravenous injection is tri-phasic[7,8]. The terminal half-life is 6–24 h after intravenous injection of conventional doses, and 30–48 h after high-dose therapy, and is a major determinant of gastrointestinal toxicity and myelosuppression. Toxicity of the gastrointestinal tract can be diminished by citrovorum rescue factor (leucovorin) given within 42 h after administration of methotrexate[6]. Monitoring methotrexate plasma concentrations may help to identify those patients at risk for increased toxicity[9]. Continuation of leucovorin rescue at standard doses (6–12 mg/m^2 every 3–6 h) for those patients with prolonged time thresholds, and augmentation of the dose for those with elevated plasma levels, may be necessary[10,11]. Intrathecal injection and drug distribution into third-space compartments such as ascites or pleural effusions may act as reservoirs, resulting in elevated plasma levels[12].

Mucositis caused by high doses of 5-FU may be associated with bloody diarrhoea in severe cases, and an associated mortality rate depending on dose, duration of injection, route of administration, and on biochemical parameters such as inborn defect of the enzyme dihydropyrimidine dehydrogenase and simultaneous modulation of 5-FU by folinic acid. Profound mucositis is more likely to occur with higher doses, shorter infusion time, intra-arterial infusion (e.g. arteria hepatica for the local chemotherapy of liver metastases), and the addition of modulators to 5-FU.

Table 2 illustrates the different toxicity profiles of 5-FU depending on the duration of infusion (bolus ($<$15 min) versus continuous infusion ($\geq$24 h)).

FACTORS INFLUENCING THE OCCURRENCE AND DEGREE OF MUCOSITIS

Patients differ markedly in the ability to tolerate a given chemotherapy regimen. Patients who developed oral toxicity within the first course of therapy often

Table 1 Cytostatic agents causing mucositis

Antimetabolites
Methotrexate (prolonged infusion), 5-FU (bolus), cytarabine, 6-mercaptopurine, thioguanine, edatrexate
Intercalating agents
Anthracyclines, bleomycin, amsacrine, actinomycin D, mitomycin C
Alkylating agents
Busulfan, cyclophosphamide, procarbazine, thiotepa
Mitotic inhibitors and topoisomerase II inhibitors
Vinca alkaloids, taxanes; etoposide (phosphate)

Table 2 Toxicity profile of 5-fluorouracil (5-FU) depending on the duration of infusion

Grade 3–4 CTC (%)	*5-FU bolus/folinic acid, day 1–5 (Mayo clinic regime)*	*5-FU continuous infusion (24 h)/folinic acid weekly*
Emesis	8	5
Diarrhoea	18	21
Mucositis	24	2
Leukopenia	29	1
Hand–foot syndrome	0	61 (53% = grade I–II; 8% = grade III–IV)

Table 3 Risk factors for mucositis

Agent/combination regimen
Mode of application
Degree of myelosuppression
  conditioning regimens for bone marrow transplantation
  conventional versus dose-intensified chemotherapy
  combination with radiotherapy, i.e. head–neck cancer patients
Mucosal irritation (trauma, faulty dental appliances)
Poor oral hygiene
Xerostomia
Patients with haematological malignancies
Age (?) (epithelial rate of proliferation)
Sex (?) (Women/5-FU)

show similar side-effects during subsequent courses unless the doses are decreased or the drugs are changed. The state of oral health, performance status and age are critical factors for the risk of complications. Young patients are reported to experience more toxicity than older patients[13]. Table 3 summarizes the known risk factors for mucositis. There is evidence that graft-versus-host disease (GvHD) can intensify oral mucositis.

INFECTIONS CAUSED BY MUCOSITIS

Infections may further complicate mucositis. About 25–50% of septicaemia in neutropenic cancer patients appears to originate from oral colonizing bacteria. Oral infections with Gram-negative organisms have decreased over time, perhaps because of both the prophylactic use of broad-spectrum antibiotics in neutropenic patients and the empirical use of intravenous antibiotics at first sign of fever. With oral bacterial infections the mucosa often has a necrotic appearance along with ulcerations. Most bacterial infections in the compromised host are caused by organisms that have been colonizing at or near the site of infection[14]. Multiple pathogens, including *Pseudomonas aeruginosa, Staphylococcus aureus*, and *Escherichia coli*, can be acquired within the oral cavity while the patient is hospitalized. Recent reports have also identified viridans streptococci as important pathogens in the neutropenic cancer patient[15].

Oral fungal infections in myelosuppressed patients are usually caused by *Candida* spp.[16]. The typical localizations of oral candidiasis are the sides and top of the tongue, the buccal and gingival mucosa, and the commissures of the lips. Fungal infections manifest as painless, wide, raised, cured-like strands or patches. Forced removal of the plaque reveals an erythematous or ulcerated mucosal surface. Diagnoses should be made by microscopic evaluation and tissue cultures.

Herpes simplex virus (HSV type I) and varicella zoster are the two most common viral pathogens causing oral infection in immunocompromised patients. The majority of HSV infections are caused by reactivation of a latent virus, whereas primary infections are extremely rare. The characteristic vesicular lesions usually rupture within a day, resulting in a diffuse ulceration. Diagnostic tests with viral cultures reveal characteristic intranuclear inclusions in the epithelial cells of stained smears.

THE PREVENTION AND TREATMENT OF MUCOSITIS

In the past two or three decades a variety of methods and agents have been introduced to prevent or to decrease the severity of mucositis in cancer patients (Table 4, adapted from Sonis[1] and from Rosenthal and Karthaus[17]); however an effective approved treatment is still lacking. Unfortunately, most trials did not include a sufficient number of patients, and they were mostly non-randomized, often non-placebo-controlled trials, with inhomogeneous patient collectives, not offering sufficient statistical power. On the other hand, validated mucositis scales have been introduced recently[18]. The most used scales, e.g. the CTC or the WHO toxicity criteria, tend to underreport or underscore mucositis[19]. The new OMAS scale (oral mucositis assessment scale) possesses a high interobserver correlation and objective mucositis scores demonstrated strong correlation with subjective symptoms (see Table 5).

Treatment approvals are primarily based on stimulation of proliferation of the basal epithelium, on surface protection of the mucosa or on the growth inhibition of microbial pathogens. However, during larger clinical trials a variety of drugs, e.g. allopurinol, sucralfate, chamomile extracts or prostaglandins, have not been proven to be successful for the prevention or therapy of mucosal injuries. It thus appears to be very difficult to recommend generally acceptable regimens for the prophylaxis and therapy of mucositis[16,20,21]. As a consequence, despite the use of several mucosal protectants, some patients may develop severe mucositis. Since there is no well-established antidote for these patients, they usually receive a local anaesthetic such as benzocaine or lidocaine to provide temporary relief of oral mucositis pain[22].

ORAL DECONTAMINATION

Chlorhexidine

Chlorhexidine digluconate (e.g. 0.12% or 0.2%), which is particularly active against Gram-positive bacteria, is often used as a mucosal protectant. Cancer

Table 4 Therapeutic agents for mucositis

	Effect on mucositis
Disinfection	
Chlorhexidine	–
H_2O_2	–
Povidone-iodine (+ others)	+ (1)
Analgesics	
Benzydamine	+ (pain↓)
Lidocaine	– (pain↓)
Indomethacin	–
Physical protectors	
Cryotherapy	+ (4)
He–Ne laser	+ (3)
Hydroxypropylcellulose	– (pain↓)
Silver nitrate	–/+
Antiulcerative drugs	
Azelastine (Vit. C/E, glutathione)	+ (1)
Pentoxifylline	–
Prostaglandins	+ (1)/– (2)
Sucralfate	+ (2)/– (4)
Metabolism modulation	
Allupurinol	– (1)/+ (1)
Glutamine	– (3)/+ (2)
β-Carotene	+
Tocopherol	+
Antiphlogistics	
Chamomile extracts	?
Other	
Amifostine	+ (3)
Immunoglobulins	+ (1)
Propantheline	+ (1)
Pilocarpine	+ (1)

Modified from Rosenthal and Karthaus[17]. +, Effective; –, no effect; figures in parentheses indicate no. of trials.

patients are instructed to rinse with 15 ml of chlorhexidine for 30 s four times daily during, and until 2 weeks after, their course of chemotherapy or irradiation. However, the degree of mucositis does not appear to be improved significantly by the drug. On the contrary, patients complain of altered taste, staining of the teeth and mouthwash discomfort. In addition the prolonged use of chlorhexidine digluconate may predispose patients undergoing bone marrow transplantation to oral colonization by Gram-negative bacilli[16,23].

A variety of other topical disinfectants are in use, e.g. hydrogen peroxide 3%, povidone iodine or cetylpyridinium chloride. However, their particular role as mucosal protectants has not been evaluated in detail[16]. The caustic agent silver nitrate (e.g. brushing with 2% $AgNO_3$ three times daily for 5 days) has also been reported to shorten the duration of mucositis. More data appear to be necessary for further recommendations[20].

Table 5 Mucositis scales

OMAS	
Location: multiple regions in oral cavity	
Erythema*	
Ulceration (pseudomembrane)†	
*0 = none, 1 = not severe, 2 = severe. †1 ≤ 1 cm^2, 2 ≤ 1–3 cm^2, 3 > 3 cm^2	
Presence of infection: local, non-oral, systemic	
CTC	
0	—
I	Painless ulcers, erythema, mild scoreness
II	Painful ulcers, oedema or ulcer, but can eat
III	Painful ulcers, oedema or ulcer, and cannot eat
IV	Requires parenteral or enteral support
WHO	
0	—
I	Painless ulcers, erythema, or mild soreness
II	Painful erythema, oedema, or ulcers but can eat solids
III	Painful erythema, oedema, or ulcers and cannot eat solids
IV	Requires parenteral or enteral support for alimentation

PTA lozenges

Lozenges containing polymyxin E, tobramycin and amphotericin B have been used to suppress oral and pharyngeal infections in cancer patients. According to the study results of Kaanders et al. the antibiotic, antifungal lozenges could successfully reduce the degree and duration of mucositis in patients with cancer of the oral cavity undergoing radio-/chemotherapy, whereas no similar effects could be observed in patients with cancers of the oropharynx[24]. More recent data confirm that these lozenges containing non-absorbable antibiotics may decrease particularly radiation-induced oral mucositis to a modest degree. However, there is still controversy as to whether these lozenges should be part of standard practice[25].

The comparison between a salt and soda mouthwash (NaCl/natrium bicarbonate) and the 'magic' mouthwash (lidocaine 0.5%, benadryl 0.25 ml (0.03%), aluminium hydroxide 14.75 ml) or chlorhexidine revealed no substantial difference in days with symptomatic mucositis[26].

A recent double-blind phase III randomized controlled trial using antimicrobial lozenges against radiation-associated mucositis in conventionally treated patients with head-and-neck cancer using a validated mucositis scoring system demonstrated no benefit[27].

Benzydamine HCl

Benzydamine HCl 0.15% as oral rinse (15 ml for 2 min) four to eight times daily before and during radiotherapy, was an effective, safe and well-tolerated regimen for prophylaxis, and was superior compared to placebo in a recently published trial[28].

Traumeel S

A small randomized controlled clinical trial in children undergoing stem cell transplantation has demonstrated that the antimicrobial and anti-inflammatory drug Traumeel S could reduce the rate of chemotherapy-induced stomatitis[29].

LOCAL VASOCONTRICTION AND INHIBITION OF SALIVARY SECRETION

Oral cryotherapy

Randomized clinical trials demonstrated that 30 min of oral cryotherapy, given at approximately the same time as the cytostatic injection of 5-FU or high-dose melphalan, can significantly inhibit the subsequent development of oral mucositis. The oral use of ice chips induces local vasoconstriction, which results in a selective reduction of drug distribution into the mucosal epithelium. This method appears to be particularly effective if drugs with a short elimination half-life are used as bolus injections[30–32].

Propantheline

Recently Oblon et al. reported that the prolonged administration of the anti-cholinergic drug propantheline (e.g. 30–60 mg every 6 h) appears to be safe and effective for the protection of the oral cavity after high-dose chemotherapy, particularly for regimens containing high-dose etoposide. According to their study results the protective effect of propantheline is restricted to the oral mucosa, whereas the severity of oesophagitis and enteritis is not influenced by this drug. The underlying mechanism of propantheline-mediated mucosal protection may be based on the decreased excretion of etoposide in saliva (via reduced saliva production) which results in lower local drug concentrations in the oral cavity. Propantheline may be an interesting candidate for supportive care in etoposide-containing regimens[33].

CHEMICAL PROTECTION OF THE MUCOSAL EPITHELIUM

Amifostine

Among the sulphydryl compounds the prodrug amifostine appears to be the most promising agent for amelioration of radiation-induced mucositis. Amifostine (WR-2721, S-2[3aminopropylamino]ethylphosphoro-thioic acid) needs to be dephosphorylated within the cells, resulting in the corresponding active metabolite WR-1065. WR-1065 is thought to exert a protective role by scavenging free radicals or by directly binding to active derivatives of antineoplastic agents, particularly platinum compounds and alkylating agents.

Amifostine has been shown to be selectively protective on normal cells because of the preferential uptake of the drug by normal cells. Alkaline phosphatase, which is a cell-surface enzyme present in high concentrations in capillaries and arterioles, is necessary for bioactivation. Tumour cells appear to contain lower levels of this enzyme based on the poor vascularization of tumour tissue. Amifostine has been approved as a protectant for the reduction of cisplatin-induced nephrotoxicity and cisplatin/cyclophosphamide-induced myelosuppression. Clinical studies regarding the protective effects of WR-2721 on oral and pharyngeal mucosa in patients receiving cancer chemotherapy are ongoing[34,35].

Granulocyte colony-stimulating factor (G-CSF)/granulocyte and monocyte colony-stimulating factor (GM-CSF)

These glycoproteins have a direct effect on endothelial cells and on keratinocytes. Both drugs are well-established protectants regarding the severity and duration of chemotherapy-induced neutropenia. Based on an open-label, phase I–II study, Gabrilove et al. suggested that the use of G-CSF resulted in significantly less mucositis in patients undergoing myelosuppressive chemotherapy for bladder cancer. However, subsequent studies did not support G-CSF or topical GM-CSF as being effective for preventing mucositis[36–39]. Therefore this question needs to be more carefully addressed in the future, before any recommendation can be given.

Sucralfate

Sucralfate is a basic aluminium salt of sucrose octasulphate that has been approved by the FDA in the USA for the treatment of duodenal ulcers. The drug forms a protective coat adhering to exposed proteins in inflamed gastroduodenal mucosa. Additionally, the local production of cytoprotective prostaglandins appears to be enhanced by sucralfate. Whereas previous data suggested that sucralfate (e.g. 1 g of sucralfate suspension four times daily as a mouth-rinse for 14 days) may be beneficial to treat chemotherapy-induced mucositis, a recent trial could not confirm the influence of the drug on the severity of chemotherapy-induced stomatitis[40–42].

Allopurinol

Clark et al. reported that an allopurinol mouthwash appeared to be successful in reducing the incidence and severity of 5-FU-induced mucositis[43]. It was speculated that the metabolite oxypurinol could impair the bioactivation of the cytotoxic drug to the corresponding phosphorylated metabolites. However, Loprinzi and colleagues could not confirm the preliminary results favouring the use of allopurinol as a mucosal protectant. There was no substantial difference in mucositis severity and frequency attributable to the allopurinol-containing mouthwash. As a consequence, allopurinol cannot be recommended as mucosal protectant in cancer patients who receive a bolus injection of 5-FU[44].

Prostaglandins: dinoprostone (prostaglandin E2) and misoprostol (PGE1)

Kührer et al. were among the first to record that topical dinoprostone might alleviate chemotherapy-induced oral mucositis[45]. Subsequent trials confirmed the special role of dinoprostone as a mucosal protectant[46]. However, these study results were not gained in a double-blind, placebo-controlled study. So far the use of prostaglandins is still controversial because clinical data are contradictory, indicating that there may be no clinical benefit, but even a more extensive oral reactivation of HSV infections in prostaglandin-treated cancer patients[47].

Plant extracts (e.g. chamomile mouthwash)

The chamomile plant, containing many different anti-inflammatory, antibacterial and spasmolytic substances, including chamazulene, bisabolole, spiroethers and flavonoids, has been used for medical purposes for centuries. It has been suggested that diluted chamomile extracts (e.g. 30 drops of a concentrate in 100 ml of water) might be advantageous to prevent chemotherapy-induced mucositis. However, according to the preliminary results of Fidler and colleagues, the use of diluted chamomile extracts could not decrease 5-FU-induced stomatits[48].

In clinical practice sage tea and diluted tormentil or myrrh tincture are often recommended for the prophylaxis of chemotherapy- or radiation-induced mucositis. In some cases these solutions may be beneficial for the patient; however, they so far represent untested topical solutions.

Vitamins

Mills was among the first to report that the administration of alpha-carotene (250 mg/day for the first 3 weeks and 75 mg/day for the next 5 weeks) as a dietary supplement might be useful to decrease the risk of grade 3–4 mucositis[49]. It has been recorded that the topical application of 1 ml of vitamin E oil (400 mg/ml) to oral lesions (e.g. twice a day for 5 days) may result in a more rapid and complete resolution of mucosal lesions[50]. However, in both cases double-blind placebo-controlled trials are still lacking.

Experimental approaches

The local application of immunoglobulins during radiation therapy of the head-and-neck area has been studied as a preventive measure for mucositis. However, no large clinical studies are yet available[45,46]. Another approach had aimed at inhibiting the cell cycling of the mucosal epithelial cells by transforming growth factor β (TGF-β3) in order to make these cells less susceptible to cytotoxic injuries. Despite this hypothetically interesting concept large-scale clinical data in cancer patients are not yet available[51].

Interleukin-11 (oprelvekin), a pleiotropic cytokine, is effective in down-relating proinflammatory mediators such as TNF-α, interleukin-1β, and nitric oxide. Results of animal studies suggest that subcutaneous injection of IL-11 favourably affects the mucositis induced by chemotherapy or radiation[52].

Another interesting cytokine in this regard is keratinocyte growth factor (KGF), a member of the fibroblast growth factors superfamily. Application of KGF results in trophic effects, and early trials in patients receiving stomatotoxic conditioning regimens with peripheral blood stem cell transplant and in patients treated for colorectal cancer have produced interesting preliminary results[53].

OTHER

Pilocarpine

The use of pilocarpine for the prevention of chemotherapy-induced oral mucositis in adult patients with cancer was evaluated in a double-blind, placebo-controlled crossover study. Thirty-two patients were included, and a total of 82 courses of chemotherapy have been reviewed. Mucositis was documented in 20 out of 41 courses in which patients were given placebo, whereas mucositis was documented in only six out of 41 courses in patients given oral pilocarpine. Therefore pilocarpine appears to be a reasonable option in the prevention of oral mucositis when given prophylactically to adult patients, and this drug should be further evaluated[54].

He–Ne laser

There are a few phase I trials published using laser effects on oral mucositis in patients receiving chemotherapy with promising results; however, prospective controlled trials including a sufficient number of patients are still lacking[55].

CONCLUSION

Undoubtedly, oral hygiene remains the most important cornerstone in patients at modest and high risk for chemo-/radiotherapy-induced stomatitis, although it is not yet standardized. Despite the use of antiseptic and cleaning mouth-rinses patients may complain of pain, and may develop local or systemic infectious diseases based on treatment-related mucosal damage. Many other strategies have been suggested to be beneficial in mucositis prophylaxis and prevention. Sufficiently powered clinical trials on the prevention and treatment of mucositis are still lacking. Internationally accepted assessment scales for measuring the severity of mucositis are of special importance for these studies. Using these scales progress will be made in the field of antitumour therapy-induced oral mucositis in the same way as haematopoietic growth factors or the treatment of chemotherapy- and radio-induced emesis and vomiting in recent years. Currently the only procedure associated with a lower frequency of chemotherapy-induced oral mucositis is the application of ice chips during application of antimetabolites with short serum half-life (cryotherapy)[56]. All other drugs, such as local chlorhexidine, sucralfate, GM-CSF, prostaglandin, allupurinol mouth-rinse, glutamine and camomile, have failed to show significant efficacy.

References

1. Sonis ST. Oral complications of cancer chemotherapy. Oncology. 2002;16:680–6.
2. Ruescher TJ, Sodeifi A, Scrivani SJ, Kaban LB, Sonis ST. The impact of mucositis on alpha-hemolytic streptococcal infection in patients undergoing autologous bone marrow transplantation for hematologic malignancies. Cancer. 1998;82:2275–81.
3. Sonis ST, Oster G, Fuchs H et al. Oral mucositis and the clinical and economic outcomes of hematopoietic stem-cell transplantation. J Clin Oncol. 2001;19:2201–5.
4. Peterman A, Cella D, Glandon G et al. Mucositis in head and neck cancer: economic and quality-of-life outcomes. J Natl Cancer Inst Monogr. 2001;29:45–51.
5. Sonis ST. Mucositis as a biological process: a new hypothesis for the development of chemotherapy-induced stomatotoxicity. Oral Oncol. 1998;34:39–43.
6. Bleyer WA. The clinical pharmacology of methotrexate: new applications of an old drug. Cancer. 1978;41:36–51.
7. Young RC, Chabner BA. An *in vivo* method for determining differential effects of chemotherapy on target tissues in animals and men. Correlation with plasmopharmacokinetics. J Clin Invest. 1973;52:92 (abstract).
8. Stoller RG, Jacobs SA, Draik JC et al. Pharmacokinetics of high-dose methotrexate (NSC-47). Cancer Chemother Rep. 1975;6:19–24.
9. Stoller RG, Hande KR, Jacobs SA, Rosenberg SA, Chabner BA. Use of plasma pharmacokinetics to predict and prevent methotrexate toxicity. N Engl J Med. 1977;297:630–4.
10. Schappner BA, Jones DG, Bertiono JR. Enzymatic cleavage of methotrexate provides a method for prevention of drug toxicity. Nature. 1972;239:395–7.
11. Jacobs WA. Clinical pharmacology; current status and therapeutic guidelines. Cancer Treat Rev. 1977;4:87–101.
12. Jacobs SA, Bleyer WA, Chabner BA, Johns DG. Altered plasma pharmacokinetics of methotrexate administered intrathecally. Lancet. 1977;1:455–6.
13. Schubert MM, Sullivan KM, Truelove EL. Head and neck complications of bone marrow transplantation. In: Petersen DE, Elias EG, Sonis ST, editors. Head and Neck Management of the Cancer Patient. Boston, MA: Nijhoff, 1986:401–27.
14. Schimpff SC. Infections in patients with cancer: overview and epidemiology. In: Moossa AR, Schimpff SC, Roxen MC, editors. Comprehensive Textbook of Oncology, 2nd edn. Baltimore, MD: Williams & Wilkins, 1991:1720–32.
15. Wingard JR. Infectious and non-infectious systemic consequences. NCI Monogr. 1990;9:21–6.
16. Peterson DE. Oral toxicity of chemotherapeutic agents. Semin Oncol. 1992;19:478–91.
17. Rosenthal C, Karthaus M. [Current approaches in prevention and therapy of chemo- and radiotherapy-induced oral mucositis]. Wien Med Wochenschr. 2001;151:53–65.
18. Sonis ST, Eilers JP, Epstein JB et al. Validation of a new scoring system for the assessment of clinical trial research of oral mucositis induced by radiation or chemotherapy. Mucositis Study Group. Cancer. 1999;85:2103–13.
19. Dodd MJ, Facione NC, Dibble SL, MacPhail L. Comparison of methods to determine the prevalence and nature of oral mucositis. Cancer Pract. 1996;4:312–18.
20. Verdi CJ. Cancer therapy and oral mucositis. Drug Safety. 1993;9:185–95.
21. Marks JE. Mucosal protectants and their application for head and neck chemoirradiation. Curr Opin Oncol. 1997;9:267–73.
22. LeVegue FG, Parzuchowski JB, Farinacci GC et al. Clinical evaluation of MCI 209, an anesthetic, film-forming agent for relief from painful oral ulcers associated with chemotherapy. J Clin Oncol. 1992;10:1963–8.
23. Foote RL, Loprinzi CL, Frank AR et al. Randomized trial of a chlorhexidine mouthwash for alleviation of radiation-induced mucositis. J Clin Oncol. 1994;12:2630–3.
24. Kaanders JHAM, Pop LAM, Uitterhoeve RJ, van Daal WAJ. Prevention of irradiation mucositis in the oral cavity and oropharynx by PTA lozenges. Int J Radiat Oncol Biol Phys.1993;27:253.
25. Okuno SH, Foote RL, Loprinzi CL et al. A randomized trial of a nonabsorbable antibiotic lozenge given to alleviate radiation-induced mucositis. Cancer. 1997;79:2193–9.
26. Dodd MJ, Dibble SL, Miaskowski C et al. Randomized clinical trial of the effectiveness of 3 commonly used mouthwashes to treat chemotherapy-induced mucositis. Oral Surg Oral Med Oral Pathol Oral Radiol Endod. 2000;90:39–47.

27. El-Sayed S, Nabid A, Shelley W et al. Prophylaxis of radiation-associated mucositis in conventionally treated patients with head and neck cancer: a double-blind, phase III, randomised, controlled trial evaluating the clinical efficacy of an antimicrobiol lozenge using a validated mucositis scoring system. J Clin Oncol. 2002;20:3956–63.
28. Epstein JB, Silverman S, Paggiarino DA et al. Benzydamine HCl for prophylaxis of radiation-induced oral mucositis. Cancer. 2001;92:875–85.
29. Oberbaum M, Yaniv I, Ben-Gal Y et al. A randomized, controlled clinical trial of the homeopathic medication Traumeel S in the treatment of chemotherapy-induced stomatitis in children undergoing stem cell transplantation. Cancer. 2001;92:684–90.
30. Dumontet C, Sonnet A, Bastion Y et al. Prevention of high-dose L-PAM-induced mucositis by cryotherapy. Bone Marrow Transplant. 1994;14;492–4.
31. Loprinzi CL, Foote RL, Michalak J. Alleviation of cytotoxic therapy-induced normal tissue damage. Semin Oncol. 1995;22:95–7.
32. Rocke LK, Loprinzi CL, Lee JK et al. A randomized clinical trial of two different durations of oral cryotherapy for prevention of 5-fluorouracil-related stomatitis. Cancer. 1993;72:2234–8.
33. Oblon DJ, Paul SR, Oblon MB, Malik S. Propantheline protects the oral mucosa after high-dose ifosfamide, carboplatin, etoposide and autologous stem cell transplantation. Bone Marrow Transplant. 1997;20:961–3.
34. Foster-Nora J, Siden R. Amifostine for protection from antineoplastic drug toxicity. Am J Health Syst Pharm. 1997;54:787–800.
35. Hartmann JT, von Vangerow A, Fels LM et al. A randomized trial of amifostine in patients with high-dose VIC chemotherapy plus autologous blood stem cell transplantation. Br J Cancer. 2001;84:313–20.
36. Gabrilove JL, Jakubowski A, Scher H et al. Effect of G-CSF on neutropenia and associated morbidity due to chemotherapy for transitional-cell carcinoma of the urothelium. N Engl J Med. 1988;318:1414–22.
37. Pettengell R, Gurney H, Radford JA et al. G-CSF to prevent dose-limiting neutropenia in non-Hodgkin's lymphoma: a randomized controlled trial. Blood. 1992;80:1430–6.
38. Hejna M, Kostler WJ, Raderer M et al. Decrease of duration and symptoms in chemotherapy-induced oral mucositis by topical GM-CSF: results of a prospective randomised trial. Eur J Cancer. 2001;37:1994–2002.
39. Sprinzl GM, Galvan O, de Vries A et al. Local application of granulocyte–macrophage colony-stimulating factor (GM-CSF) for the treatment of oral mucositis. Eur J Cancer. 2001;37:2003–9.
40. Pfeiffer P, Madesn EL, Hansen O, May O. Effect of prophylactic sucralfate suspension on stomatitis induced by cancer chemotherapy: a randomized, double-blind cross-over study. Acta Oncol. 1990;29:171–3.
41. McGinnis WL, Loprinzi CL, Buskirk SJ et al. Placebo-controlled trial of sucralfate for inhibiting radiation-induced esophagitis. J Clin Oncol. 1997;15:1239–43.
42. Loprinzi CL, Ghosh C, Comoriano J et al. Phase III controlled evaluation of sucralfate to alleviate stomatitis in patients receiving fluorouracil-based chemotherapy. J Clin Oncol. 1997;15:1235–8.
43. Clark PI, Slevin ML. Allopurinol mouthwash and 5-fluorouracil induced oral toxicity. Eur J Surg Oncol. 1985;11:267–8.
44. Loprinzi CL, Cianflone SG, Dose AM et al. A controlled evaluation of an allopurinol mouthwash as prophylaxis against 5-fluorouracil-induced stomatitis. Cancer. 1990;65:1879–82.
45. Kührer I, Kuzmits R, Linkesch W, Ludwig H. Topical PGE2 enhances healing of chemotherapy-associated mucosal lesions. Lancet. 1986;1:623.
46. Porteder H, Rausch E, Kment G et al. Local prostaglandin E2 in patients with oral malignancies undergoing chemo- and radiotherapy. J Cranio-Maxill Facial Surg. 1988;16:371–4.
47. Labar B, Mrsic M, Pavletic Z et al. Prostaglandin E2 for prophylaxis of oral mucositis following bone marrow transplantation. Bone Marrow Transplant. 1993;11:379–82.
48. Fidler P, Loprinzi CL, O'Fallon JR et al. Prospective evaluation of a chamomile mouthwash for prevention of 5-FU-induced oral mucositis. Cancer. 1996;77:522–5.
49. Mills EED. The modifying effect of beta-carotene on radiation and chemotherapy induced oral mucositis. Br J Cancer. 1988;57:416–17.
50. Wadleigh RG, Redman RS, Graham ML et al. Vitamin E in the treatment of chemotherapy-induced mucositis. Am J Med. 1992;92:481–4.
51. Sonis ST, Lindquist L, Van Vugt A et al. Prevention of chemotherapy-induced ulcerative mucositis by transforming growth factor β3. Cancer Res. 1994;54:1135–8.

52. Trepicchio WL, Ozawa M, Walters IB et al. Interleukin-11 therapy selectively downregulates type I cytokine proinflammatory pathways in psoriasis lesions. J Clin Invest. 1999;104:1527–37.
53. Booth D, Potten CS. Protection against mucosal injury by growth factors and cytokines. JNCI Monogr. 2001;29:16–20.
54. Awidi A, Homsi U, Kakail RI et al. Double-blind, placebo-controlled cross-over study of oral pilocarpine for the prevention of chemotherapy-induced oral mucositis in adult patients with cancer. Eur J Cancer. 2001;37:2010–14.
55. Wong SF, Wilder-Smith P. Pilot study of laser effects on oral mucositis in patients receiving chemotherapy. Cancer J. 2002;8:247–54.
56. Worthington HV, Clarkson JE. Prevention of oral mucositis and oral candidiasis for patients with cancer treated with chemotherapy: Cochrane systematic review. J Dent Educ. 2002;66:903–11.

13
Neutropenic enterocolitis, enteric infections

M. GORSCHLÜTER, T. SAUERBRUCH and A. GLASMACHER

INTRODUCTION

The number of neutropenic patients is continuously on the rise, which results in a proportional increase of infections during neutropenia. Among these infections the most common forms are fever of unknown origin (FUO), pneumonia and bacteraemia. However, the gastrointestinal tract is also often affected, due to the mucosal toxicity of cytotoxic agents used for the treatment of haematological malignancies. These agents result in a considerable destruction of anatomical barriers against infections. Together with the acquired insufficiency of humoral and cellular immunity, these patients are prone to severe enteric infections.

This chapter attempts to give an overview of the diagnostic criteria, the incidence and the therapy of neutropenic enterocolitis. Furthermore, available evidence on specific enteric infectious agents that cause infections in these patients is reviewed.

ABDOMINAL INFECTIONS IN PATIENTS WITH HAEMATOLOGICAL MALIGNANCIES

Abdominal infections in neutropenic patients are among those with the highest case fatality rate, especially in patients with acute leukaemia and aggressive cytostatic chemotherapy[1–3]. Typical forms of these infections are – most importantly – neutropenic enterocolitis, cholecystitis and hepatosplenic candidiasis. The reported incidence rates for neutropenic enterocolitis vary between 2.6% and 32.2% with the highest incidence in children and a mortality rate of 50% and more[2–4]. Prospectively evaluated incidence rates for neutropenic enterocolitis, cholecystitis and *Clostridium difficile*-associated diarrhoea were not available until recently. Unfortunately many studies do not use standardized diagnostic criteria or prospective screening methods such as abdominal sonography.

Table 1 Diagnostic criteria for neutropenic enterocolitis (all three criteria must be present)

Presence of fever (axillary temperature > 38.0°C or rectal temperature > 38.5°C) *and*
at least one clinical symptom at the abdomen (abdominal pain, diarrhoea) *and*
demonstration of bowel wall thickening by ultrasonography or computed tomography

DIAGNOSIS OF NEUTROPENIC ENTEROCOLITIS

In accordance with several studies in the literature we defined diagnostic criteria for neutropenic enterocolitis (Table 1)[6].

INCIDENCE OF SEVERE ABDOMINAL INFECTIONS IN NEUTROPENIC PATIENTS WITH HAEMATOLOGICAL MALIGNANCIES

In a retrospective study in our hospital, from 1991 until 1997, 553 courses of myelosuppressive chemotherapy in patients with acute leukaemia or aggressive non-Hodgkin's lymphomas were evaluated. Among these patients 16 severe abdominal infections occurred[5]. Thirteen of these were shown to be a neutropenic enterocolitis, and three were cholecystitis. This corresponds to a frequency of 1.8% (10/553) of all neutropenic episodes in patients with acute leukaemia following myelosuppressive chemotherapy. Five of these patients (50%) died due to neutropenic enterocolitis.

In our prospective survey (which included sonography screening) an incidence of 6.5% (4/62) for neutropenic enterocolitis (NEC) and 4.8% (3/62) for cholecystitis was found[6]. Two of four identified patients with NEC died. In the literature an incidence of up to 30% has been reported, but most studies were of poorer methodological quality[7–9]. Many reports came from paediatric centres but it is unclear whether the disease occurs more often in children[4,9].

CAUSES AND CLINICAL COURSE OF ABDOMINAL INFECTIONS IN NEUTROPENIC PATIENTS

In our two series of the six patients with cholecystitis one died from pneumonia and another from simultaneous neutropenic enterocolitis and septic shock. The other four patients could be managed conservatively during the period of neutropenia, and cholecystectomy was performed after that in two patients[5,6]. Among all 17 patients with enterocolitis and haematological malignancies a pathogen was detected in 12 (70.6%) patients (Table 2). Likewise others have seen bacteraemia in 28–82% of cases[1] and have isolated *Escherichia coli*, *Klebsiella pneumoniae*, *Pseudomonas aeruginosa*, *Enterobacter*, staphylococci and streptococci, as well as *Candida* spp.[8–10].

Nine of the 17 patients in our combined series died; one from pneumonia and eight under the clinical form of septic shock. Three of these patients had a surgical procedure (left-sided colostomy one, explorative laparotomy one, appendectomy one). All of the patients who had surgical procedures survived. Survival

Table 2 Microbiota responsible for neutropenic enterocolitis in our series (modified, from refs 5 and 6)

Escherichia coli: 4
Pseudomonas aeruginosa: 1
Streptococcus mitis: 1
P. mirabilis: 1
Clostridium difficile: 1
Candida glabrata: 1
Candida krusei: 1
Aspergillus fumigatus: 1
Cytomegalovirus: 1

was, however, connected with the procedure in only one patient who had suffered a mechanical ileus and was relieved by colostomy[5,6].

DIAGNOSTIC PROCEDURES FOR NEUTROPENIC ENTEROCOLITIS

Sonography is more and more being recognized as a valuable diagnostic tool in the diagnosis of neutropenic enterocolitis. Demonstration of intestinal wall thickening is generally accepted as a criterion for a clinical diagnosis[5,6,8,11], and reflects the pathological characteristics of neutropenic enterocolitis such as extensive mucosal and submucosal oedema with occasional bleeding, ulceration and necrosis[12].

Cartoni et al. showed that intestinal wall thickening is an important negative prognostic factor[11]. Our prospective study did not show any intestinal wall thickening in 29 asymptomatic patients who were screened for comparison, and in only one episode with symptoms that did not fulfil our clinical criteria for neutropenic enterocolitis[6]. The maximal intestinal wall thickness ranged between 5.8 mm (ileum) and 23.6 mm (caecum) with 11.3 mm (descending colon) and 16.7 mm (caecum) in two other patients.

Some authors have requested histopathological confirmation for the diagnosis of NEC[1]. Although there is a typical histological pattern[7,10,12], we do not think that a biopsy or resection should be required or attempted to confirm the diagnosis of NEC. As will be discussed later, surgery (and endoscopy) are difficult in these neutropenic and thrombocytopenic patients. Furthermore, as empirical antibiotic therapy is a necessity, therapeutic consequences from the biopsy are improbable (with rare exceptions, e.g. diagnosis of cytomegalovirus).

Laboratory tests are non-specific and cannot help to make the diagnosis. Intensive surveillance of these patients is, however, necessary as electrolyte imbalances, coagulation disorders, etc. frequently occur. Standard diagnostic work-up should include frequent blood cultures and stool cultures.

We conclude that intestinal wall thickening is characteristic for neutropenic enterocolitis and that sonography is a useful bedside screening method that quickly gives important information concerning the nature of the abdominal infection. A computed tomography scan may be useful if sonography does not allow a complete examination of the abdomen for technical reasons such as severe meteorism, or if surgery is considered.

CLOSTRIDIUM DIFFICILE INFECTIONS IN NEUTROPENIC PATIENTS

In another retrospective survey in our hospital we analysed 61 independent episodes with *Clostridium difficile*-associated diarrhoea in 53 patients[13]. These episodes were found upon analysis of 875 neutropenic episodes in patients with acute leukaemia and myelosuppressive chemotherapy. Therefore the incidence of *Clostridium difficile*-associated diarrhoea (CDAD) per neutropenic episode was 7.0% (61/875). Only 35 (57.4%) of 61 patients with CDAD had previously received intravenous antibiotic therapy. Twenty-five episodes (41.9%) occurred during oral antibiotic prophylaxis with cotrimoxazole and colistin. No case of bacteraemia by *Clostridium difficile*; no complication such as toxic megacolon, intestinal obstruction or intestinal perforation; and no deaths directly related to *Clostridium difficile* occurred.

OTHER SPECIFIC AGENTS CAUSING ENTERIC INFECTIONS

Only in three of 1185 stool specimens that were taken in a 6-year period in our hospital from neutropenic patients with acute leukaemia, and were tested for *Salmonella*, *Shigella*, *Yersinia* or *Campylobacter*[14], did cultures reveal a microorganism being searched for. All three cultures came from the same patient, who suffered from food-borne infection by *Salmonella enteritidis*. So in total only one of 371 episodes of diarrhoea could be attributed to these infectious agents; therefore the incidence of an infection by these agents was 0.32% per patient in the period analysed. The incidence of these infections per course of myelosuppressive therapy was 0.14% (1/731).

In our prospective study only one patient had an infection from these agents (*Campylobacter jejuni*) which led to the incidence of 1.6% (1/62 neutropenic episodes)[14]. Cytomegalovirus infections or reactivations leading to enteritis were also very rare in our patients, which included only very few patients after allogeneic bone marrow transplantation. We could prove a CMV colitis in only one of 553 patients during the 6-year retrospective period, and in no patient during the prospective study period[5,6].

MORTALITY OF NEUTROPENIC ENTEROCOLITIS

The mortality of neutropenic enterocolitis is very high, and ranges in the literature from 3% to more than 50%[2,11,15]. In our studies we observed a mortality rate of 52.9% (9/17), which is well in line with the published data. This is also in line with reports from the literature[11]. Our studies also show that the outcome depends on the recovery of neutrophils.

THERAPY OF NEUTROPENIC ENTEROCOLITIS AND CHOLECYSTITIS

The usual treatment is conservative and non-surgical, especially because the difficulties of surgery in neutropenic thrombocytopenic septic patients are considerable. The antibiotic treatment should include a good activity against *Pseudomonas aeruginosa*, *Escherichia coli* and anaerobes. In our clinic this comprised mostly piperacillin–tazobactam monotherapy, with good clinical results and a low induction of resistance. The question whether metronidazole should be added when NEC is detected even in the absence of *Clostridium difficile* is still not solved. On the one hand broad-spectrum antibiotics such as piperacillin–tazobactam have a very good activity against anaerobic bacteria; on the other hand sufficient intraluminal activity is achieved only with metronidazole, as the drug is excreted with the bile.

Empirical antifungal therapy is also strongly recommended in accordance with international guidelines, and in the view of three proven and one suspected invasive fungal infections among 17 patients with NEC in our combined series[5,6]. According to current available evidence conventional amphotericin B, liposomal amphotericin B or itraconazole should be used.

Contrary to the clear indication for antibiotic therapy, controversy still surrounds the role of surgery. Clear indications for an operation are, of course, intestinal perforation, complete intestinal obstruction and peritonitis. It is very doubtful, however, whether resection of inflamed bowel, in the absence of these complications, is beneficial[2,15]. We would not attempt this in neutropenic and thrombocytopenic patients with acute leukaemia and NEC. However, as the clinical signs of an acute abdomen may occur to some extent in these patients, the decision to perform or to withhold an exploratory laparotomy is quite difficult, and needs considerable clinical experience as well as intense cooperation between haematologists and surgeons.

The same problem applies also to patients with acute cholecystitis in neutropenia. We could manage four of six patients with antibiotic therapy, and could defer cholecystectomy to the period after recovery of haematopoiesis.

CONCLUSION

Neutropenic enterocolitis is a rare, but for diseased patients frequently fatal, infectious syndrome that occurs most frequently in patients with haematological malignancies and under myelosuppressive chemotherapy. Typical infectious agents causing these syndromes are Gram-negative bacteria and fungi. Classical bacterial enteric pathogens (*Salmonella*, *Shigella*, *Yersinia* and *Campylobacter* spp.) and viruses are found only rarely in these infections. Treatment is primarily conservative with empirical broad-spectrum antibiotic therapy, and surgery is reserved for vital indications such as complete intestinal obstruction or intestinal perforation.

Adequate awareness by clinicians is necessary, and may be supported by sonography screening of patients showing clinical symptoms, especially the combination of fever and abdominal pain. Our proposed criteria for the diagnosis of neutropenic enterocolitis could help to define the syndrome, detect complications earlier, and to initiate specific treatments early (especially antibiotic coverage for anaerobes).

Further research, particularly prospective studies, is urgently needed, and should concentrate on the analysis of risk factors, the possibility of prophylaxis and the development of more successful therapeutic concepts that could lower the high mortality rate in this severe infection.

Acknowledgement

The studies reported in this review were supported by Leukämie-Initiative Bonn e.V. and Deutsche José Carreras Leukämie-Stiftung e.V.

References

1. Bavaro MF. Neutropenic enterocolitis. Curr Gastroenterol Rep. 2002;4:297–301.
2. Wade DS, Nava HR, Douglass HO Jr. Neutropenic enterocolitis. Clinical diagnosis and treatment. Cancer. 1992;69:17–23.
3. Mower WJ, Hawkins JA, Nelson EW. Neutropenic enterocolitis in adults with acute leukemia. Arch Surg. 1986;121:571–4.
4. Shamberger RC, Weinstein HJ, Delorey MJ, Levey RH. The medical and surgical management of typhlitis in children with acute nonlymphocytic (myelogenous) leukemia. Cancer. 1986;57:603–9.
5. Gorschlüter M, Glasmacher A, Hahn C et al. Severe abdominal infections in neutropenic patients. Cancer Invest. 2001;19:669–77.
6. Gorschlüter M, Marklein G, Hofling K et al. Abdominal infections in patients with acute leukaemia: a prospective study applying ultrasonography and microbiology. Br J Haematol. 2002;117:351–8.
7. Quigley MM, Bethel K, Nowacki M, Millard F, Sharpe R. Neutropenic enterocolitis: a rare presenting complication of acute leukemia. Am J Hematol. 2001;66:213–19.
8. Gomez L, Martino R, Rolston KV. Neutropenic enterocolitis: spectrum of the disease and comparison of definite and possible cases. Clin Infect Dis. 1998;27:695–9.
9. Sloas MM, Flynn PM, Kaste SC, Patrick CC. Typhlitis in children with cancer: a 30-year experience. Clin Infect Dis. 1993;17:484–90.
10. Katz JA, Wagner ML, Gresik MV, Mahoney DH Jr, Fernbach DJ. Typhlitis: an 18-year experience and postmortem review. Cancer. 1990;65:1041–7.
11. Cartoni C, Dragoni F, Micozzi A et al. Neutropenic enterocolitis in patients with acute leukemia: prognostic significance of bowel wall thickening detected by ultrasonography. J Clin Oncol. 2001;19:756–61.
12. Moir DH, Bale PM. Necropsy findings in childhood leukaemia, emphasizing neutropenic enterocolitis and cerebral calcification. Pathology. 1976;8:247–58.
13. Gorschlüter M, Glasmacher A, Hahn C et al. *Clostridium difficile* infection in patients with neutropenia. Clin Infect Dis. 2001;33:786–91.
14. Gorschlüter M, Hahn C Ziske C et al. Low frequency of enteric infections by *Salmonella, Shigella, Yersinia* and *Campylobacter* in patients with acute leukemia. Infection. 2002;30:22–5.
15. Alt B, Glass NR, Sollinger H. Neutropenic enterocolitis in adults. Review of the literature and assessment of surgical intervention. Am J Surg. 1985;149:405–8.

14
Management of chemotherapy-induced diarrhoea

M. SCHULTZ, J. SCHÖLMERICH and F. KULLMANN

INTRODUCTION

Bowel dysfunction, such as diarrhoea and constipation, can be a disturbing side-effect in chemotherapy that may result not only in significant physical and emotional distress for the patients and caregivers[1], but also in diminished therapy efficacy due to dose limitations and treatment interruptions. Chemotherapy-induced diarrhoea (CID) first became apparent during clinical studies on the combination of 5-fluorouracil (5-FU) with leucovorin, and furthermore with irinotecan in the treatment of metastatic colorectal carcinoma[2,3].

Dose intensity is a function of dose and frequency of administration, and is defined as the amount of drug delivered per unit of time (e.g. mg/m^2 per week). In a retrospective study a clear relation between dose intensity and outcome in patients with breast cancer was shown in both adjuvant and metastatic settings[4,5]. The consequences of chemotherapy dose delay and reduction have been clearly shown by Norton[6] based on the 'Gompertzian' kinetics of the growth of human tumours, meaning that the proportion of cells killed is greater when the number of cells is low, but also that the tumour re-growth rate is higher when cell numbers decrease. Furthermore, in animal studies, using an osteosarcoma mouse model, it became evident that a reduction in dose intensity had a great impact on cure rate, without affecting the rate of complete remission[7].

Diarrhoea is much less common than constipation, particularly due to the use of opioid analgesia, but occurs in up to 4–10% in patients with advanced cancer[8–10]. However, besides leucocytopenia, thrombocytopenia, and granulocytopenia, CID is considered one of the main dose-limiting toxicities associated with chemotherapy agents, especially in treatment regimens for colorectal cancer, and can even be life-threatening[10]. It should not be forgotten that common causes of diarrhoea affecting the general population, such as infectious agents, etc., can be present in the patient with cancer disease who is undergoing chemotherapy.

Clinical assessment and diagnostic evaluations should include these common aetiologies. In a recent retrospective study approximately 52% of patients experienced diarrhoea of grades 3 or 4, leading to modifications in their chemotherapy regime, such as dose reductions, delays in therapy, discontinuations of therapy or even multiple changes[11]. Due to the nature of agents used in chemotherapy, and the susceptibility of the intestinal mucosa, there are many reagents causing diarrhoea (Table 1); however, the risk of CID is significantly higher for regimens with newer chemotherapeutic agents such as antimetabolites (e.g. 5-fluorouracil, methotrexate) and topoisomerase-I inhibitors (e.g. irinotecan, topotecan) and anthracyclins (e.g. doxorubicin and daunorubicin). Reported incidences range from 23% to 44%[12], in some studies even as high as 60–70%[13–16] for irinotecan, and from 4% to 10% with low-dose 5-FU[17] up to 16–26% for high-dose 5-FU in combination with leucovorin[18–21]. Although dose reduction and schedule modification have reduced morbidity and mortality, the results of several large trials that compared different dosing schedules of 5-FU and different combinations of regimens with leucovorin have shown that CID remains an issue of concern[22–25].

In order to achieve and maintain remission in colorectal cancer disease, adjuvant chemotherapy and abdominal radiation are often used, but are known to increase the potential for the development of CID[26].

The pathogenesis of CID is not fully understood, but is probably the result of combined mechanisms; therefore it remains difficult to provide guidelines for the treatment and/or prevention of CID. This chapter will review the scientific literature, and will try to provide a pathophysiologically based approach to the clinical management of CID.

Table 1 Common chemotherapy agents causing CID

Agent	*Dose-limiting side-effects*
Capecitabine	Diarrhoea, nausea, hand–foot syndrome
Cisplatin	Tumour resistance, myelosuppression, gastrointestinal side-effects
Cytosine arabinoside	Stomatitis, mucositis
Cyclophosphamide	Alopecia, dermatitis, neuropathy, nausea, vomiting, diarrhoea
Daunorubicin	Gastrointestinal side-effects, delayed cardiotoxicity
Docetaxel	Myelosuppression, enteritis, diarrhoea, fluid retention
Doxorubicin	Alopecia, dermatitis, neuropathy, nausea, vomiting, diarrhoea
5-Fluorouracil	Diarrhoea
Interferon	Nausea, vomiting
Irinotecan	Cholinergic syndrome, nausea, vomiting, delayed diarrhoea, myelosuppression
Methotrexate	Tumour resistance
Oxaliplatin	Neuropathy, gastrointestinal side-effects
Topotecan	Cholinergic syndrome, nausea, vomiting, delayed diarrhoea, myelosuppression

PATHOPHYSIOLOGICAL CONSIDERATIONS

In the healthy patient, digestion and the elimination of waste products occur in the gastrointestinal tract. When food reaches the stomach a complex system of muscle and nerve activities stimulates gastric, pancreatic, and biliary secretions. After a few hours the stomach contents are passed into the small bowel. About 10 L of fluids are passed daily into the small bowel, not only from oral intake (approximately 2 L/day), but also due to secretion of the various intestinal glands (7–8 L/day). Here the villi are responsible for absorption of most electrolytes, water, iron, calcium, folate, fats, carbohydrates, proteins, and sugars. In 6–9 h the small bowel contents, including 1–1.5 L/day fluid, are passed into the large intestine, where bacterial vitamin synthesis and further fluid absorption take place, before formed stool is passed through the rectum. Normally, 98% of the intestinal fluid is passively absorbed by the small and large intestine due to the osmotic gradient from the intraluminal to the extraluminal compartment (Figure 1). The amount of absorption is determined by the amount of electrolytes and other osmotically relevant luminal contents, such as carbohydrates and amino acids. In contrast, sodium and chloride are actively transported, but the large intestine lacks carriers for the transport of sugars and amino acids. These substances are degraded or utilized for protein synthesis by colonic anaerobic bacteria.

Destruction of mucosal integrity due to chemotherapy and/or radiation can lead to a diminished absorption of fluids followed by an imbalance of electrolytes.

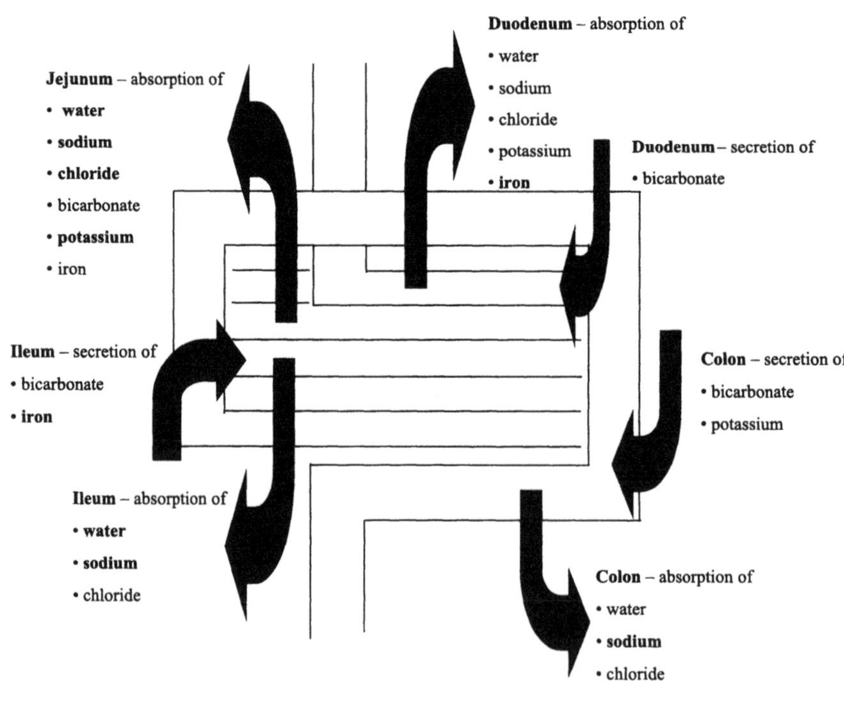

Figure 1 Absorption and resorption of fluids and electrolytes throughout the gastrointestinal tract

The underlying pathomechanism is not fully understood. The intestinal mucosa is characterized by a very fast cell turnover of less than 2 days. Using animal models it was shown that chemotherapeutic agents affect dose-dependently the mitotic cell turnover of intestinal epithelial cells. Radiation leads initially to an increased intestinal motility[27,28], followed by a decrease in length of the intestinal villi, decreased mitotic rate and influx of inflammatory cells[29].

All the disorders that cause diarrhoea in the general medical setting can be observed in advanced cancer patients. Chronic diarrhoea can be caused by infections, inflammatory bowel disease, irritable bowel disease, dietary alterations, laxative abuse, endocrine disorders, neoplasms, malabsorption syndromes, surgery, or radiation, while CID is usually considered acute, because it is associated with a drug reaction. Other causes of acute diarrhoea include infections, dietary alterations, inflammatory bowel diseases, intestinal ischaemia, or faecal impaction (Table 2).

There are four basic pathophysiological mechanisms of chronic and acute diarrhoea:

1. Osmotic diarrhoea occurs when there is an increased amount of hyperosmolar solutes in the gut lumen (e.g. carbohydrates, enteral feeding solutions, blood).
2. Secretory diarrhoea results from the inhibition of normal ion absorption or ion secretion. This might occur due to a loss or destruction of epithelial cells (e.g. due to infections, inflammatory processes and chemotherapy).
3. Dysmotility diarrhoea is caused by an alteration in normal gut motility, and can be hypo or hyper, both leading to an increased number of bowel movements.
4. Exudative diarrhoea is caused by a disruption of the intestinal mucosa secondary to inflammation (e.g. chemotherapy). As a result proteins, mucus, and blood are released into the intestines and promote the development of diarrhoea as in radiation colitis, inflammatory bowel disease, or colonic neoplasms.

The pathophysiological mechanisms of CID seem to be multilayered and of the secretory (exudative) type, caused by an imbalance between absorption and

Table 2 Common causes of diarrhoea in cancer patients

Directly cancer-associated causes	Partial bowel obstruction, enterocolic fistula, villous adenoma, endocrine-induced hypersecretion of serotonin, gastrin, calcitonin, vasoactive intestinal prostaglandins
Cancer-related causes	Melaena, steatorrhoea, faecal impaction, anxiety
Coincidental	Infectious gastroenteritis, diverticulitis, inflammatory bowel disease, irritable bowel disease, scleroderma, hyperthyroidism, diabetes mellitus, lactose deficiency, dietary fibre, dietary bowel stimulants
CID	Refer to Table 1
Post-surgery	Involving gastrectomy, pancreatectomy, blind-loop syndrome, ileal resection, palliative bypass operation
Radiotherapy	Of abdomen, pelvis, lower spine
Adjuvant therapy of symptoms and concomitant medication	Laxatives, antacids, NSAID, enteral nutritional supplements, metoclopramide, theophylline, caffeine, alcohol

secretion, mainly affecting the function of the small bowel. The loss of intestinal epithelium, inflammation, disturbed intestinal motility, and superficial necrosis of the bowel occurs as a result of acute damage to the intestinal mucosa from certain chemotherapeutic agents. The inflammatory process and necrosis can furthermore stimulate secretion of fluids and electrolytes directly and allow the symptoms to persevere[30–32]. Different chemotherapy agents can cause varying degrees of diarrhoea due to their mechanism of action.

The highest incidences of CID have been reported with regimens including 5-FU, leucovorin and CPT-11; therefore we will discuss the pathophysiological mechanisms of these agents, leading to diarrhoea, in more detail.

5-Fluorouracil/leucovorin

The combination of 5-FU and leucovorin increases the intracellular concentration of 5-FU[33], and therefore antineoplastic effects[2], but aggravates dose-limiting side-effects including alopecia, hyperpigmentation, photosensibilization, and bloody diarrhoea. These side-effects seem not only to be dose-related but also dependent on the type of administration (bolus, continuous infusion) and the length of the treatment-free intervals between cycles[34]. However, in a recent phase III study comparing weekly folinic acid (FA) and high-dose 5-FU with monthly 5-FU/FA (days 1–5) toxicity was moderate and roughly comparable with the exception of a higher occurrence of hand–foot syndrome in the weekly treatment regime. No difference was seen in gastrointestinal side-effects[35].

Several investigations have been undertaken to characterize the underlying pathomechanisms of 5-FU-related diarrhoea. Clinical and histological studies revealed that high-dose 5-FU-based chemotherapy not only induces a colitis[36], but may also involve the upper small intestinal tract. Microscopic studies of the stool all remained negative, including *Clostridium difficile* and its toxins A and B, but the endoscopic appearance of the intestinal mucosa of the lower intestinal tract ranged from normal to colitis-like alterations, including diffuse erythema and microulcerations. Endoscopy of the upper intestinal tract revealed similar alterations, ranging from close-to-normal mucosa to isolated ulcerations. Histological examination showed destruction of the superficial mucosa and crypts in the sense of apoptosis of the epithelium[37]. This is accompanied by increased small intestinal permeability and therefore diminished intestinal absorption[38].

Recent work relates the occurrence of severe side-effects to a genetic defect involving the 5-FU metabolism[39–41]. The incidence of this defect is approximately 1%. The enzyme dihydropyrimidine dehydrogenase (DPD) catalyses the rate-limiting step of 5-FU biotransformation to yield the first inactive metabolite 5-fluoro-5,6-dihydrouracil[42]. Decreased DPD activity leads to delayed inactivation of 5-FU and therefore accumulation over an extended period of time. Abnormally low values of DPD activity in the liver, but not in peripheral mononuclear cells, was associated with the occurrence of major adverse effects after 5-FU treatment[43–45]. In a recent study it was demonstrated that in five patients who experienced severe gastrointestinal toxicities (i.e. grade 3–4 diarrhoea or stomatitis), marked changes in 5-FU pharmacokinetic parameters were observed in contrast to subjects who tolerated the treatment well[45].

These observations support the hypothesis that the level of systemic elimination of 5-FU is responsible for the occurrence of severe toxicity[39,46,47].

In summary treatment with 5-FU/leucovorin shows a direct effect on the intestinal mucosa, affecting both the upper and lower intestinal tract. This might be aggravated due to delayed 5-FU elimination due to a genetic defect, involving 5-FU metabolism.

Irinotecan (CPT-11)

The clinical use of CPT-11 at higher dosages is associated with a significant incidence of diarrhoea, with great inter-patient variability. Characteristically, the episodes of the developing diarrhoea can be divided temporally into two parts, first appearing about 1 h after the injection of CPT-11, sometimes even interrupting the infusion, and later about 3–4 days following chemotherapy. In order to treat this interfering side-effect one has to fully understand the underlying pathomechanisms and the varying efficacy of conventional antidiarrhoeal agents[13,15,16,48].

One possible explanation is that CPT-11 itself has anticholinesterase activity[49], which causes acute diarrhoea by stimulating intestinal contractility, and impairs normal intestinal mucosal absorptive and secretory functions[50,51]. Other possible mechanisms might include structural and functional damage to the intestinal tract that results from the mitotic inhibitory activity of the active metabolite of CPT-11, SN-38, which is thought to be relevant to the antitumour activity of CPT-11[52,53]. Furthermore, it has been reported that CPT-11/SN-38 have absorption characteristics of weak basic drugs, suggesting that alkalization of the intestinal lumen might reduce reabsorption[54–56]. Additionally, stasis of stools containing the chemotherapeutic compounds is thought to induce damage to the intestinal mucosa[57–59]. Oral alkalization and control of defaecation appear useful in preventing the dose-limiting side-effects of CPT-11[60].

A further explanation for the severe CID has been given by Takasuna et al.[61]. Following administration, a major proportion of CPT-11 is hydrolysed to form the active metabolite SN-38, which is further conjugated in part in the liver to SN-38 glucuronide (SN38-glu) and then excreted into the bile together with the remaining SN-38 and CPT-11[52,62,63]. SN38-glu is processed back to SN-38 by β-glucuronidase, an enzyme provided by the intestinal microflora in the caecum[52]. Since patients with diminished or no UDP-glucuronyltransferase activity, such as in those with either Crigler-Najjar syndrome I or Gilbert's syndrome[62,64], it became apparent that the glucuronyltransferase, which forms SN38-glu, plays a major role in the developing diarrhoea[65]. Experimental inhibition of the β-glucuronidase activity in the intestinal microflora of rats by antibiotics markedly ameliorated the diarrhoea and reduced the histological damage to the caecum in rats[61]. This was confirmed by the use of neomycin in cancer patients receiving CPT-11[66]. This shows that the microflora in the large intestine is capable of having a significant effect in the development of diarrhoea induced by CPT-11; however, CPT-11 and SN-38 have no direct antibacterial activity.

In summary, CPT-11-induced diarrhoea might be two-fold. The initial episode of diarrhoea might be due to direct anticholinergic activity by the compound itself. Regarding the delayed episode of diarrhoea it is thought that CPT-11 and/or its active metabolite SN-28 primarily affects the rapidly proliferating crypt cells, which delays the onset of diarrhoea associated with the functional impairment of villus epithelial cells, similar to those shown by other anticancer agents[58,67]. The increasing severity of the diarrhoea following repeated injections of CPT-11[58] might be due to the effect of increasing concentrations of β-glucuronidase in the intestinal microflora, as shown above, and since inhibitors of DNA topoisomerase-I inhibitors are highly cycle-phase specific[68], the severity of CPT-11/SN-38-induced intestinal cytotoxicity may be influenced more by the duration of exposure of cells to these substances than by their concentrations[52].

Other mechanisms

Neutropenic enterocolitis is a well-known complication of chemotherapy in children and adults with leukaemia, and is observed in approximately 25%[69]. Some chemotherapeutic agents such as paclitaxel, 5-FU, and irinotecan are associated with neutropenia and CID. The occurrence of neutropenic enterocolitis related to treatment with different chemotherapeutic combinations is rare, but encompasses 5-FU, and should therefore be considered in the clinical work-up of CID[70].

DIAGNOSTIC APPROACH

Diagnosis of the cause of diarrhoea is often a difficult challenge due to the number of clinical entities that produce this symptom in advanced cancer patients. Acute diarrhoea can be defined as the passage of a greater number of stools of decreased form compared with the normal, lasting for less than 14 days but more than 4 days[71]. However, the situation in patients receiving chemotherapy might differ from that in otherwise healthy patients. The assessment of associated diseases can provide important clues concerning the aetiology. Due to the underlying consuming disease, and the ongoing, often immunosuppressive therapy, prompt assessment of patients with suspected CID is critical. As a result of the persistent loss of fluids and electrolytes, life-threatening dehydration, renal insufficiency, electrolyte imbalances, cardiovascular complications and collapse might occur. Early recognition and treatment can prevent the morbidity and mortality associated with CID. The most commonly used assessment tool is the National Cancer Institute Common Toxicity Criteria for Grading the Severity of Diarrhoea[108].

Table 3 National Cancer Institute Common Toxicity Criteria for Grading the Severity of Diarrhoea[72]

	Grade 0	*Grade 1*	*Grade 2*	*Grade 3*	*Grade 4*
Number of stools	Normal	2–3/day	4–6/day	7–9/day	>10/day
Symptoms	None	None	Moderate cramping and nocturnal stools but not interfering with normal activities	Severe cramping and incontinence, interfering with daily activity	Grossly bloody diarrhoea and need for parenteral support

Other critical factors that should be assessed are onset and duration of diarrhoea; current medication or other therapy, including radiation to the pelvis for malignancies of the urogenital tract or prostate; dietary and fluid intake; weight loss; measures taken to control the diarrhoea; and any other symptoms such as nausea and vomiting, lightheadedness, vertigo, or fevers. From the clinical point of view the suspicion of partial obstruction should be raised in cases with sudden diarrhoea after a period of constipation. Previous surgical procedures or the presence of foul-smelling or oily stools suggests fat malabsorption.

The physical examination is also an important element in the assessment of diarrhoea[73], and should include vital signs. Strict indications for medical evaluation include dehydration, defined as dry mucous membranes, decreased skin turgor, decreased urination, and tachycardia, sometimes accompanied by hypotension. Often the critically ill patient seems confused, disorientated, and drowsy. The abdominal assessment should include examination for tenderness, guarding, rebound tenderness, distension, organomegaly, and hyperactive or hypoactive bowel sounds. With a rectal examination one should look for stool occult blood and faecal impaction. Laboratory studies should include a white blood count, a metabolic panel including sodium and potassium serum levels to detect any electrolyte imbalances, BUN for possible renal impairment and dehydration. In selected cases radiographic studies with plain abdominal films for signs of an ileus should be obtained. Occasionally computed tomography can be helpful in patients with suspected bowel obstruction (Figure 2).

Fever is usually a finding associated with an invasive pathogen that produces intestinal inflammation. Only these cases should be studied for aetiological agents, and many will benefit from antimicrobial therapy[74]. The potential for neutropenia that leads to sepsis is increased in patients who receive 5-FU and CPT-11. Thus, fever in these patients might indicate the high risk of sepsis. Although diarrhoea, occurring during ongoing chemotherapy is often caused by the compound itself, as described above, an infectious cause should be considered and evaluated before commencing treatment. According to the guidelines of the American Gastroenterological Association and the American Society of Gastrointestinal Endoscopy, immunocompromised patients with diarrhoea should receive a limited evaluation of stool microbiology followed by full evaluation only for patients failing to respond to specific or symptomatic treatment. A more detailed evaluation is not indicated in view of the low yield for treatable aetiological agents when an expensive work-up is undertaken (Figure 2)[71].

TREATMENT CONSIDERATIONS

In former times the treatment of CID was focused mainly on symptomatic management of diarrhoea, such as the reduction of frequency of stools, skin impairment, the discomfort associated with frequent diarrhoea and the prevention of dehydration during the recovery of the acutely damaged intestinal mucosa[75]. Diarrhoea can be managed successfully with a variety of general, specific, and symptomatic therapeutic strategies. In this review we will concentrate on the management of CID. Traditional pharmacological management of CID has included mainly non-specific agents. For patients who are refractory to

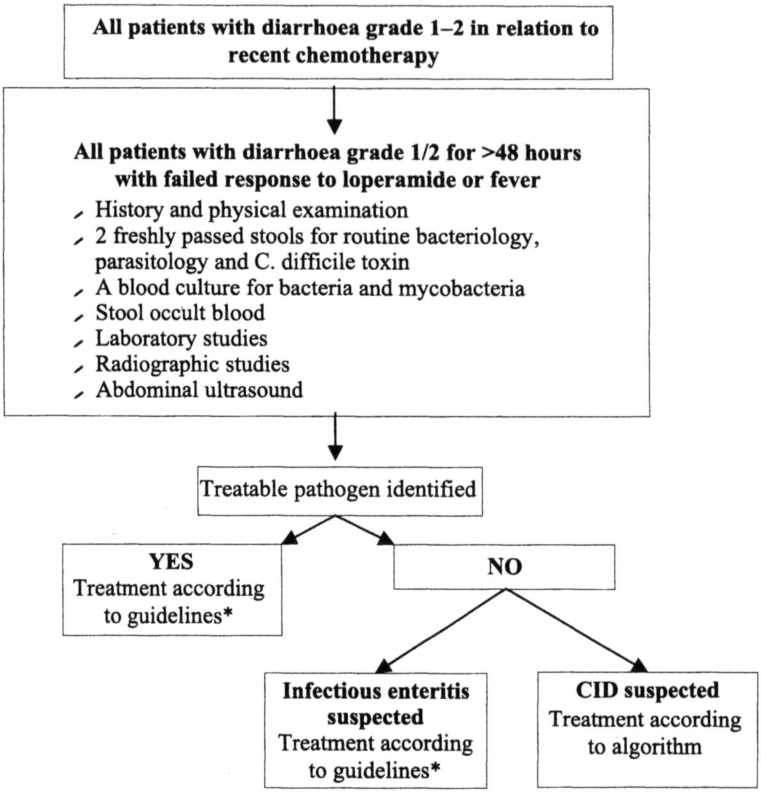

Figure 2 Assessment algorithm of patients with low-grade diarrhoea (grade 0–2)[71]

non-specific therapy there are more sophisticated, specific therapeutic agents available.

As a first step before any aetiological considerations, clinical signs of dehydration imply the need for intravenous or, if possible, oral hydration and hospitalization.

Non-specific symptomatic therapy

Non-pharmacological approaches

Diarrhoea in patients with advanced cancer can often be eased with some general dietary modifications. Initial management should include avoidance of foods and medicines that aggravate CID. Lactose-free and low-fat diets could be beneficial in patients with malabsorption, especially in the short bowel syndrome. For patients with prominent dumping, frequent small, dry meals, high in protein and potassium and low in carbohydrates, such as the BRAT diet (bananas, rice, peeled apples and dry white bread) may be useful[76]. Other dietary recommendations include avoiding cold and/or spicy meals, milk and dairy products, fatty meat, fish, fruit juices, coffee and alcohol[77].

Pharmacological approaches

Opioid receptors, especially μ and δ, are well represented on gut smooth muscle, either in the myenteric plexus or submucous plexus. These receptors influence intestinal motility and, as a consequence, secretion. Opioids, such as loperamide and diphenoxylate, produce many effects at different levels of the intestinal tract, including increased ileocaecal tone, decreased small intestinal and colon peristalsis with increased electrolyte and water absorption, and impaired defaecation reflex by increased anal sphincter pressure[9]. Loperamide, the most commonly used drug in patients with CID, is able to reduce ileal calcium fluxes with an activity independent of its opioid effect, and it does not cross the blood barrier. It shows the highest antidiarrhoeal–analgesic ratio among the opioid-like agents, and is the drug of choice due to its few adverse effects. The dose should be titrated against effects and can exceed 12 mg per day. In the initial phase I studies of CPT-11, CID appeared to be dose-limiting at 350 mg/m^2[3,48,78]. To reduce the incidence of CID in CPT-11 treatment regimens, high-dose loperamide therapy was adopted as part of the standard protocol for the management of CPT-11-induced diarrhoea[79]. This allowed the escalation of the CPT-11 dose used in clinical trials[80] to 500–600 mg/m^2 with an incidence of CID of 9–30%[12,81].

Specific therapy and experimental approaches

These strategies to control diarrhoea include the use of specific treatments that act directly on the epithelial cells to reduce excess secretion and promote salt and water absorption. Most have been tested on a very limited number of patients, and can therefore not be recommended for use outside specialty centres.

Octreotide

The rationale for the use of octreotide in CID is based on its direct effects on somatostatin receptors on epithelial cells in the gastrointestinal tract. Octreotide inhibits gastrointestinal motility, gastric and pancreatic exocrine secretion, the release of several gastrointestinal peptides and splanchnic blood flow. On the other hand, it stimulates sodium and chloride absorption, decreases the secretion of fluids and electrolytes, and increases intestinal transit time, thereby promoting increased absorption of fluids and electrolytes[82–84]. If the CID cannot be controlled by dietary modifications or the use of high-dose opioids, such as loperamide, alleviation of diarrhoea, induced by cisplatin compounds[85], 5-FU[86–88], and irinotecan[89] has been reported with octreotide. Few controlled trials to treat and/or prevent diarrhoea, induced by 5-FU/leucovorin have been published with contradictory results[90]. There is evidence for a beneficial prophylactic and therapeutic use of octreotide, superior to loperamide (95% *vs* 15%)[85,88,91].

Octreotide has also been successfully used in the management of irinotecan-induced diarrhoea after failure of loperamide treatment. In a phase I trial, 23/37 patients receiving irinotecan experienced grade III–IV diarrhoea and were treated with loperamide; 13 patients received octreotide after loperamide failed to control diarrhoea and exhibited with a high response rate of 92%[89].

Dosage recommendations range between 100 and 150 μg subcutaneous octreotide up to three times daily. However, since ocrtreotide is only the backup choice for the treatment of CID, the patient should be admitted into hospital and kept under close observation.

Glutamine

The non-essential amino acid glutamine is an important nutrient of the gastrointestinal tract and is necessary to protect the structure and function of the gut[92,93]. Toxicity of chemotherapy can lead to reduced food intake and glutamine deficiency. In experimental studies and clinical trials the beneficial effect of glutamine supplementation on chemotherapy-induced mucositis and mucosal atrophy, and nutritional status was demonstrated[94–96]. In a recent study 24 patients treated with 5-FU/leucovorin for metastatic colorectal cancer were randomized to receive glycyl-L-glutamine parenterally (14–22 g glutamine/day). In the glutamine group a significant reduction in mucositis and ulcerations in the gastric and duodenal mucosa was documented, but there were no significant differences in the incidence and severity of clinical side-effects, including CID[96]. The underlying effect might be the reduction of changes in intestinal absorption and intestinal permeability induced by 5-FU/leucovorin[38].

A positive effect of glutamine supplementation to prevent CID has also been published for CPT-11. In five patients oral glutamine supplementation successfully prevented late-onset irinotecan-related diarrhoea after loperamide failure[97].

Oral alkalization

It has been reported that CPT-11 and its active metabolite SN-38 have absorption characteristics of weak basic drugs, suggesting that alkalization of the human intestine might reduce reabsorption and therefore prevent side-effects[98]. In a recent clinical pilot study the combination of oral alkalization (sodium bicarbonate, ursodeoxycholic acid, magnesium oxide, basic water per os) and control of defaecation with a 5-HT3 receptor antagonist appeared to be useful in preventing the dose-limiting side effects of CDP-11[60].

Anticholinergic agents

CPT-11/SN-38-induced diarrhoea may occur at two time-points in relation to the infusion of the chemotherapeutic agent. While the second episode of diarrhoea generally appears 6 days following treatment, and is fairly hard to control, the first setting is observed immediately after CPT-11 infusion and is short-lasting. This phenomenon is related to the early metabolism of CPT-11 into SN-38 (see above) and can be controlled by the administration of 0.25 mg atropine subcutaneously or intravenously[99].

Thalidomide

Thalidomide has known antineoplastic and immunomodulary properties by inhibiting the synthesis of (tumour necrosis factor) TNF-α, increasing T-helper-2 cell functions and decreasing T-helper-1 cell functions. That leads to an up-regulation of (interleukin) IL-4 and IL-5 and a down-regulation of (interferon) IFN-γ and IL-12. For these anti-inflammatory effects thalidomide undergoes a revival in the treatment of chronic inflammatory bowel disease. A pilot study of combination therapy with thalidomide and irinotecan for metastatic colorectal cancer was performed by Govindarajan et al. In an interim analysis, in 8/9 patients receiving thalidomide (400 mg/day), no gastrointestinal toxic effects from irinotecan were seen[100].

Budenoside

While corticosteroids might be beneficial in terminally ill cancer patients to boost appetite and physical well-being, the use of the locally (terminal ileum/colon) effective budenoside has produced contradictory results. While there are reports of successful treatment of CID due to irinotecan and 5-FU with budenoside[101], a recent European multicenter trial had to be terminated (personal communication).

Neomycin

As described above, CPT-11 needs to be hydrolysed by a carboxylesterase to form the active metabolite SN-38. SN-38 is then metabolized by UDP-glucuronosyltransferase to form the inactive form SN-38-glu. It was recently suggested from animal models that β-glucuronidases, provided by the intestinal microflora in the caecum, play a major role in the development of CID by irinotecan, by mediating hydrolysis of SN-38-glu back into the active and toxigenic metabolite SN-38. Inhibition of the β-glucuronidase activity from the intestinal microflora with the administration of penicillin and streptomycin led to a decrease of the luminal SN-38 concentration with amelioration of CID[61]. In a clinical trial seven patients with grade > 2 CID following irinotecan chemotherapy were given neomycin 1 g/day. Diarrhoea was ameliorated in 6/7 patients, but neomycin had no effect on haematological toxicity[66].

α_2-*Adrenoceptor antagonists*

The clinical efficacy of 5-HT3-receptor antagonists such as granisetron, ondansetron and tropisetron was first established in chemotherapy-induced emesis. The antiemetic effect is mediated by the simultaneous action at peripheral and central receptors, while obstipation occurs as a side-effect due to the serotonin antagonism[102]. Ondansetron prolongs colon transit time and leads to an increase of fluid absorption and a reduction of bowel movement frequency[103,104]; however, there is insufficient clinical evidence to recommend 5-HT3-receptor antagonists for the treatment of CID.

Various therapeutic agents with specific indications

Bile acid-binding resins such as cholestyramine could be efficacious in controlling diarrhoea due to ileal surgery with reduction of absorptive surface[105]. Aspirin has been reported to be effective in post-radiotherapy diarrhoea[106] due to its reduction in prostaglandin synthesis.

RECOMMENDATIONS FOR THE MANAGEMENT OF CHEMOTHERAPY-INDUCED DIARRHOEA

Guidelines for the treatment of CID as discussed by a panel of experts were published some years ago[107]. Since then new clinical trials have been performed with different approaches to manage CID, and further understanding was achieved in regard to the pathophysiological aspects of CID.

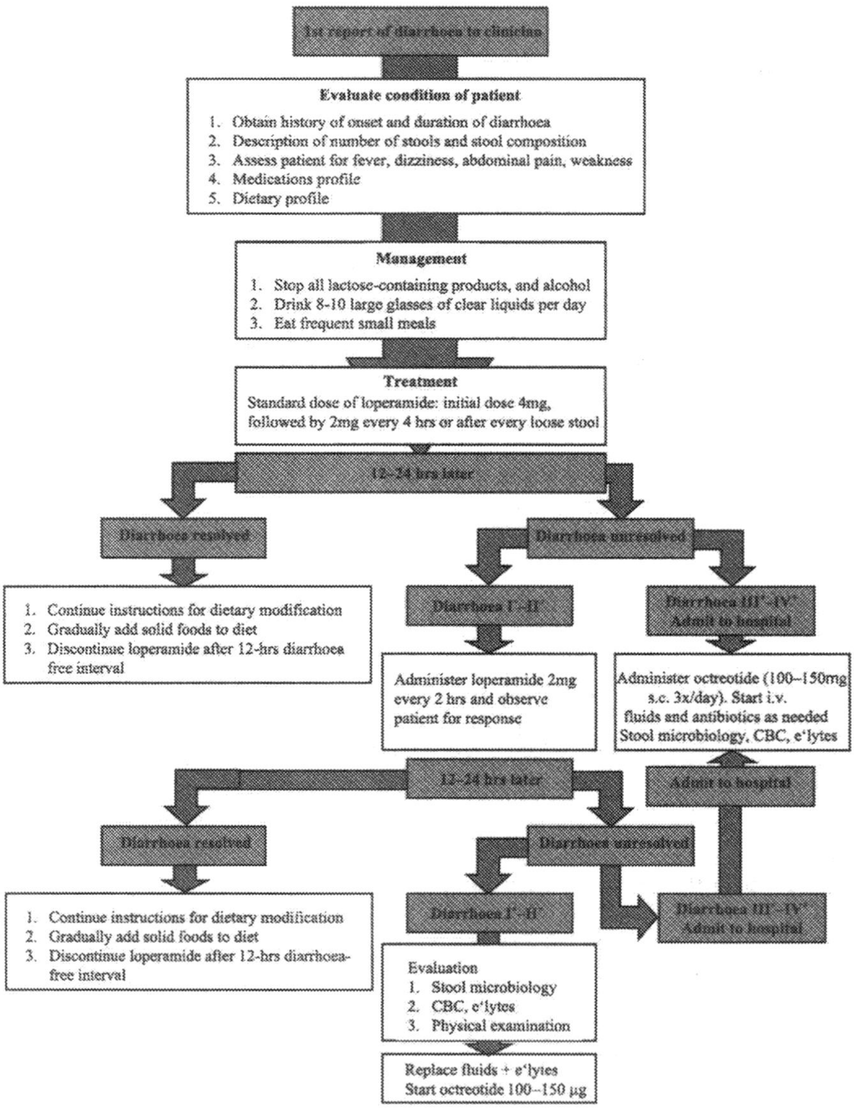

Figure 3 Recommended guidelines for the treatment of CID[26]

Initially the patient needs to be assessed for the severity of the presenting symptoms. Mainly the possibility of an infectious origin should be ruled out, before treatment for CID can be commenced (Figure 3).

Low-grade diarrhoea (grade 0–2)

Dietary modifications should be recommended to the patient before non-specific pharmacological therapy with loperamide is initiated. Treatment should be commenced with 4 mg loperamide, continued with 2 mg every 2 h until diarrhoea has ceased, but not exceeding 48 h due to the considerable risk of developing a paralytic ileus. If diarrhoea persists for more than 48 h, despite loperamide, the possibility of a cause not related to chemotherapy should be assessed, if necessary by stool cultures, abdominal ultrasound, and radiographic studies. Only then should treatment with octreotide be considered, with doses between 100 and 150 μg subcutaneously up to three times daily until diarrhoea resolves. Additionally, the patient should be admitted to the hospital for intravenous rehydration.

High-grade diarrhoea (grade 3–4)

The patient with CID grade 3 and 4 diarrhoea is in great discomfort and needs urgent hospital admission and evaluation. Loperamide is of limited effect in the treatment of severe diarrhoea. However, in the case of irinotecan-induced diarrhoea, a trial with high-dose loperamide (4 mg every 2 h) might be recommended for 24 h. Otherwise, octreotide 150 μg subcutaneously three times daily should be given until diarrhoea resolves. In the case of fever and/or neutropenia, adequate antibiotic therapy should accompany octreotide.

In the event that diarrhoea continues, despite octreotide, few clinical data are available for further management. Careful dose escalations by 50 μg have been reported to be beneficial in cases of 5-FU-induced diarrhoea[107]. In any case chemotherapy should be interrupted until diarrhoea has ceased.

References

1. Engelking C, Wickham R, Iwamoto R. Cancer-related gastrointestinal symptoms: dilemmas in assessment and management. Dev Support Cancer Care. 1996;1:3–10.
2. Petrelli N, Douglass HO Jr, Herrera L et al. The modulation of fluorouracil with leucovorin in metastatic colorectal carcinoma: a prospective randomized phase III trial. Gastrointestinal Tumor Study Group. J Clin Oncol. 1989;7:1419–26.
3. de Forni M, Bugat R, Chabot TT et al. Phase I and pharmacokinetic study of the camptothecin derivative irinotecan, administered on a weekly schedule in cancer patients. Cancer Res. 1994;54:4347–54.
4. Hryniuk WM, Bush H. The importance of dose intensity in chemotherapy of metastatic breast cancer. J Clin Oncol. 1984;2:1281–8.
5. Hryniuk WM, Figueredo A, Goodyear M. Applications of dose intensity to problems in chemotherapy of breast and colorectal cancer. Semin Oncol. 1987;14(Suppl.):3–11.
6. Norton L. Evolving concepts in the systemic drug therapy of breast cancer. Semin Oncol. 1997;24(Suppl.):S10-3–S10-10.
7. Skipper H. Data and analyses having to do with the influence of dose intensity and duration of treatment (single drugs and combination) on lethal toxicity and therapeutic response of experimental treatment. Southern Research Institute 1986; Booklet 13.
8. Regnard CFB, Tempest S. A Guide to Symptom Relief in Advanced Cancer. Manchester: Haigh & Hockland, 1992.

9. Sykes NP. Constipation and diarrhoea. In: Doyle D, Hanks GW, MacDonald N, editors Oxford Textbook of Palliative Medicine. Oxford: Oxford Medical, 1993:299–310.
10. Levy MH. Constipation and diarrhoea in cancer patients. Cancer Bull. 1991;43:412–22.
11. Arbuckle RB, Huber SL, Zacker C. The consequences of diarrhoea occurring during chemotherapy for colorectal cancer: a retrospective study. Oncologist. 2000;5:250–9.
12. Rothenberg ML, Eckhardt JR, Kuhn JG et al. Phase II trial of irinotecan in patients with progressive or rapidly recurrent colorectal cancer. J Clin Oncol. 1996;14:1128–35.
13. Fukuoka M, Niitani H, Suzuki A et al. A phase II study of CPT-11, a new derivative of camptothecin, for previously untreated non-small-cell lung cancer. J Clin Oncol. 1992;10:16–20.
14. Rothenberg ML, Kuhn J, Burris HA et al. A phase I and pharmacotrial of CPT-11 in patients with refractory solid tumors. Proc Am Soc Clin Oncol. 1992;11:113.
15 .Matsuda N, Fukuoka M, Kudoh S et al. Phase I and pharmacologic study of irinotecan in combination with cisplatin for advanced lung cancer. Br J Cancer. 1993;68:777–82.
16. Shimada Y, Yoshino M, Wakui A et al. Phase II study of CPT-11, a new camptothecin derivative, in metastatic colorectal cancer. CPT-11 Gastrointestinal Cancer Study Group. J Clin Oncol. 1993;11:909–13
17. Moertel C, Fleming TR, Macdonald JS et al. Levamisole and fluorouracil for adjuvant therapy of resected colon carcinoma. N Engl J Med. 1990;322:352–8.
18. Ardalan B, Chua L, Tian EM et al. A phase II study of weekly 24-hour infusion with high-dose fluorouracil with leucovorin in colorectal carcinoma. J Clin Oncol. 1991;9:625–30.
19. Wolmark N, Rockette H, Mamounas E et al. Clinical trial to assess the relative efficacy of fluorouracil and leucovorin, fluorouracil and levamisole, and fluorouracil, leucovorin, and levamisole in patients with Dukes' B and C carcinoma of the colon: results from National Surgical Adjuvant Breast and Bowel Project C-04. J Clin Oncol. 1999;17:3553–9.
20. Wein A, Riedel C, Bruckl W et al. Weekly 24-h infusion of high-dose 5-fluorouracil (5-FU) with folinic acid (FA) in adjuvant therapy of colon cancer. Z Gastroenterol. 2001;39:153–6.
21. Porschen R, Bermann A, Loffler T et al. Fluorouracil plus leucovorin as effective adjuvant chemotherapy in curatively resected stage III colon cancer: results of the trial adjCCA-01. J Clin Oncol. 2001;19:1787–94.
22. Leichman CG, Fleming TR, Muggia FM et al. Phase II study of fluorouracil and its modulation in advanced colorectal cancer: a Southwest Oncology Group study. J Clin Oncol. 1995;13:1303–11.
23. International Multicentre Pooled Analysis of Colon Cancer Trials (IMPACT) Investigators. Efficacy of adjuvant fluorouracil and folinic acid in colon cancer. Lancet. 1995;345:939–44.
24. Laufman LR, Bukowski RM, Collier MA et al. A randomized, double-blind trial of fluorouracil plus placebo versus fluorouracil plus oral leucovorin in patients with metastatic colorectal cancer. J Clin Oncol. 1993;11:1888–93.
25. Macdonald JS. Adjuvant therapy for colon cancer. Cancer J Clin. 1997;47:243–56.
26. Wadler S, Benson AB III, Engelking C et al. Recommended guidelines for the treatment of chemotherapy-induced diarrhoea. J Clin Oncol. 1998;16:3169–78.
27. Fernandez-Banares F, Villa S, Esteve M et al. Acute effects of abdominopelvic irradiation on the orocecal transit time: its relation to clinical symptoms, and bile salt and lactose malabsorption. Am J Gastroenterol. 1991;86:1771–7.
28. Erickson BA, Otterson MF, Moulder JE, Sarna SK. Altered motility causes the early gastrointestinal toxicity of irradiation. Int J Radiat Oncol Biol Phys. 1994;28:905–12.
29. Sher ME, Bauer J. Radiation-induced enteropathy. Am J Gastroenterol. 1990;85:121–8.
30. Baskerville A, Batter-Hatton D. Intestinal lesions induced experimentally by methotrexate. Br J Exp Pathol. 1977;58:663–9.
31. de Roy van Zuidewijn DB, Schillings PH, Wobbes T, Hendriks T, de Boer HH. Morphometric analysis of the effects of antineoplastic drugs on mucosa of normal ileum and ileal anastomoses in rats. Exp Mol Pathol. 1992;56:96–107.
32. Milles SS, Muggia AL, Spiro HM. Colonic histologic changes induced by 5-fluorouracil. Gastroenterology. 1962;43:391–9.
33. Rustum YM, Cao S, Zhang Z. Rationale for treatment design: biochemical modulation of 5-fluorouracil by leucovorin. Cancer J Sci Am. 1998;4:12–18.
34. Germ JL. Fluorinated pyrimidines. In: Chatsner BA, Collins JM, editors. Cancer Chemotherapy Principles and Practice. Philadelphia: J.B. Lippincott, 1990:197–200.
35. Weh HJ, Zschaber R, Braumann D et al. A randomized phase III study comparing weekly folinic acid (FA) and high-dose 5-fluorouracil (5-FU) with monthly 5-FU/FA (days 1–5) in untreated patients with metastatic colorectal carcinoma. Onkologie. 1998;21:403–7.

36. Poon MA, O'Connell MJ, Wieand HS et al. Biochemical modulation of fluorouracil with leucovorin: confirmatory evidence of improved therapeutic efficacy in advanced colorectal cancer. J Clin Oncol. 1991;9:1967–72.
37. Madisch A, Wiedbrauck F, Marquard F, Stolte M, Hotz J. 5-fluorouracil-induced colitis – a review based upon consideration of 6 cases. Z Gastroenterol. 2002;40:59–66.
38. Daniele B, Secondulfo M, De Vivo R et al. Effect of chemotherapy with 5-fluorouracil on intestinal permeability and absorption in patients with advanced colorectal cancer. J Clin Gastroenterol. 2001;32:228–30.
39. Tuchman M, Stoeckeler JS, Kiang DT, O'Dea RF, Ramnaraine ML, Mirkin BL. Familial pyrimidinemia and pyrimidinuria associated with severe fluorouracil toxicity. N Engl J Med. 1985;313:245–9.
40. Harris BE, Carpenter JT, Diasio RB. Severe 5-fluorouracil toxicity secondary to dihydropyrimidine dehydrogenase deficiency. A potentially more common pharmacogenetic syndrome. Cancer. 1991;68:499–501.
41. van Kuilenburg AB, Vreken P, Abeling NG et al. Genotype and phenotype in patients with dihydropyrimidine dehydrogenase deficiency. Hum Genet. 1999;104:1–9.
42. Allegra CJ. Dihydropyrimidine dehydrogenase activity: prognostic partner of 5-fluorouracil? Clin Cancer Res. 1999;5:1947–9
43. Harris BE, Song R, Soong SJ, Diasio RB. Relationship between dihydropyrimidine dehydrogenase activity and plasma 5-fluorouracil levels with evidence for circadian variation of enzyme activity and plasma drug levels in cancer patients receiving 5-fluorouracil by protracted continuous infusion. Cancer Res. 1990;50:197–201.
44. Stephan F, Etienne MC, Wallays C, Milano G, Clergue F. Depressed hepatic dihydropyrimidine dehydrogenase activity and fluorouracil-related toxicities. Am J Med. 1995;99:685–8.
45. Di Paolo A, Danesi R, Falcone A et al. Relationship between 5-fluorouracil disposition, toxicity and dihydropyrimidine dehydrogenase activity in cancer patients. Ann Oncol. 2001;12:1301–6.
46. Takimoto CH, Lu ZH, Zhang R et al. Severe neurotoxicity following 5-fluorouracil-based chemotherapy in a patient with dihydropyrimidine dehydrogenase deficiency. Clin Cancer Res. 1996;2:477–81.
47. Milano G, Etienne MC. Individualizing therapy with 5-fluorouracil related to dihydropyrimidine dehydrogenase: theory and limits. Ther Drug Monit. 1996;18:335–40.
48. Abigerges D, Chabot GG, Armand JP, Herait P, Gouyette A, Gandia D. Phase I and pharmacologic studies of the camptothecin analog irinotecan administered every 3 weeks in cancer patients. J Clin Oncol. 1995;13:210–21.
49. Kawato Y, Tsutomi T, Akahane K, Sekiguchi M, Sato K. Inhibitory effect of CPT-11, a derivate of camptothecin, on acetylcholinesterase, and its binding ability to acetylcholine receptors. Clin Report. 1990;24:7407–12.
50. Takasuna K, Kasai Y, Yamashita N et al. General pharmacological study on CPT-11. Clin Report. 1990;24:7413–33.
51. Takasuna K, Kasai Y, Kitano Y et al. Study on the mechanisms of diarrhoea induced by a new anticancer camptothecin derivate, irinotecan hydrochloride (CPT-11), in rats. Folia Pharmacol Jpn. 1995;105:447–60.
52. Kaneda N, Nagata H, Furuta T, Yokokura T. Metabolism and pharmacokinetics of the camptothecin analogue CPT-11 in the mouse. Cancer Res. 1990;50:1715–20.
53. Kawato Y, Aonuma M, Hirota Y, Kuga H, Sato K. Intracellular roles of SN-38, a metabolite of the camptothecin derivative CPT-11, in the antitumor effect of CPT-11. Cancer Res. 1991;51:4187–91.
54. Charman WN, Porter CJ, Mithani S, Dressman JB. Physiochemical and physiological mechanisms for the effects of food on drug absorption: the role of lipids and pH. J Pharm Sci. 1997;86:269–82.
55. Bugaut M. Occurrence, absorption and metabolism of short chain fatty acids in the digestive tract of mammals. Comp Biochem Physiol B. 1987;86:439–72.
56. Kobayashi K, Bouscarel B, Matsuzaki Y, Ceryak S, Kudoh S, Fromm H. pH dependent uptake of irinotecan and its active metabolite, SN-38, by intestinal cells. Int J Cancer. 1999;83:491–6.
57. Atsumi R, Okazaki O, Hakusui H. Pharmacokinetics of SN-38 [(+)-(4S)-4,11-diethyl-4,9-dihydroxy-1H-pyrano[3′,4′:6,7]-indolizino[1,2-b]quinoline-3,14(4H,12H)-dione], an active metabolite of irinotecan, after a single intravenous dosing of 14C-SN-38 to rats. Biol Pharm Bull. 1995;18:1114–9.

58. Araki E, Ishikawa M, Iigo M, Koide T, Itabashi M, Hoshi A. Relationship between development of diarrhoea and the concentration of SN-38, an active metabolite of CPT-11, in the intestine and the blood plasma of athymic mice following intraperitoneal administration of CPT-11. Jpn J Cancer Res. 1993;84:697–702.
59. Kobayashi K, Shinbara A, Kamimura M et al. Irinotecan (CPT-11) in combination with weekly administration of cisplatin (CDDP) for non-small-cell lung cancer. Cancer Chemother Pharmacol. 1998;42:53–8.
60. Takeda Y, Kobayashi K, Akiyama Y et al., Prevention of irinotecan (CPT-11)-induced diarrhoea by oral alkalization combined with control of defecation in cancer patients. Int J Cancer. 2001;92:269–75.
61. Takasuna K, Hagiwara T, Hirohashi M et al. Involvement of beta-glucuronidase in intestinal microflora in the intestinal toxicity of the antitumor camptothecin derivative irinotecan hydrochloride (CPT-11) in rats. Cancer Res. 1996;56:3752–7.
62. Iyer L, King CD, Whithington PF et al. Role of uridine diphosphate glucuronosyltransferase isoform 1A1 in the glucuronidation of its active metabolite (SN-38) in human liver microsomes. J Clin Invest. 1998;101:847–54.
63. Atsumi R, Suzuki W, Hakusui H. Identification of the metabolites of irinotecan, a new derivative of camptothecin, in rat bile and its biliary excretion. Xenobiotica. 1991;21:1159–69.
64. Wassermann EL, Myara A, Lokiec F et al. Severe CPT-11 toxicity in patients with Gilbert's syndrome: two case reports. Ann Oncol. 1997;8:149–51.
65. Gupta E, Lestingi TM, Mick R, Ramirez J, Vokes EE, Ratain MJ. Metabolic fate of irinotecan in humans: correlation of glucuronidation with diarrhoea. Cancer Res. 1994;54:3723–5.
66. Kehrer DF, Sparreboom A, Verweij J et al. Modulation of irinotecan-induced diarrhoea by cotreatment with neomycin in cancer patients. Clin Cancer Res. 2001;7:1136–41.
67. Taminiau JA, Gall DG, Hamilton JR. Response of the rat small-intestine epithelium to methotrexate. Gut. 1980;21:486–92.
68. Del Bino G, Skierski JS, Darzynkiewicz Z. The concentration-dependent diversity of effects of DNA topoisomerase I and II inhibitors on the cell cycle of HL-60 cells. Exp Cell Res. 1991;195:485–91.
69. Varki AP, Armitage JO, Feagler JR. Typhlitis in acute leukemia: successful treatment by early surgical intervention. Cancer. 1979;43:695–7.
70. Kronawitter U, Kemeny NE, Blumgart L. Neutropenic enterocolitis in a patient with colorectal carcinoma: unusual course after treatment with 5-fluorouracil and leucovorin – a case report. Cancer. 1997;80:656–60.
71. DuPont HL and the Practice Parameters Committee of the American College of Gastroenterology. Guidelines in acute infectious diarrhoea in adults. Am J Gastroenterol. 1997;92:1962–75.
72. Cope DG. Palliative and supportive care of advanced cancer: management of chemotherapy-induced diarrhoea and constipation. Nurs Clin N Am. 2001;36:695–707.
73. Held-Warmkessel J. Diarrhoea. In: Camp-Sorrel D, Hawkins R, editors. Clinical Manual for the Oncology Advanced Practice Nurse. Pittsburgh, PA: Oncology Nursing Press, 2000:343–50.
74. DuPont HL. Review article: Infectious diarrhoea. Aliment Pharmacol Ther. 1994;8:3–13.
75. Martz CH. Diarrhoea. In: Groenwald SL, Frogge MH, Goodman M et al., editors. Cancer Symptom Management. Boston, MA: Jones & Barlett, 1996:498–520.
76. Hogan CM. The nurse's role in diarrhoea management. Oncol Nurs Forum. 1998;25:879–86.
77. Mercadante S. Diarrhoea in terminally ill patients: pathophysiology and treatment. J Pain Symptom Manage. 1995;10:298–309.
78. Catimel G, Chabot GG, Guastalla JP et al. Phase I and pharmacokinetic study of irinotecan (CPT-11) administered daily for three consecutive days every three weeks in patients with advanced solid tumors. Ann Oncol. 1995;6:133–40.
79. Abigerges D, Armand JP, Chabot GG et al. Irinotecan (CPT-11) high-dose escalation using intensive high-dose loperamide to control diarrhoea. J Natl Cancer Inst. 1994;86:446–9.
80. Merrouche Y, Extra JM, Abigerges D et al. High dose-intensity of irinotecan administered every 3 weeks in advanced cancer patients: a feasibility study. J Clin Oncol. 1997;15:1080–6.
81. Conti JA, Kemeny NE, Saltz LB et al. Irinotecan is an active agent in untreated patients with metastatic colorectal cancer. J Clin Oncol. 1996;14:709–15.
82. Cooper JC, Williams NS, King RFGJ, Barker MCJ. Effects of a long-acting somatostatin analogue in patients with severe ileostomy diarrhoea. Br J Surg. 1986;73:128–31.

83. Dueno MI, Baj JC, Santangelo WC, Krejs J. Effect of sandostatin analog on water and electrolyte transport and transit time in human small bowel. Dig Dis Sci. 1987;32:1092–6.
84. Fried M. Octreotide in the treatment of refractory diarrhoea. Digestion. 1999;60:42–6.
85. Cascinu S, Fedeli A, Fedeli SL, Catalano G. Control of chemotherapy-induced diarrhoea with octreotide. Oncology. 1994;51:70–3.
86. Kennedy P, Pressant CA, Blayney D, Wiseman C, King M, Gala K. Sandostatin therapy for chemotherapy and radiotherapy-induced diarrhoea. Proc Am Soc Clin Oncol. 1993;9:324.
87. Cascinu S, Fedeli A, Fedeli SL, Catalano G. Control of chemotherapy-induced diarrhoea with octreotide in patients receiving 5-fluorouracil. Eur J Cancer. 1992;28:482–3.
88. Cascinu S, Fedeli A, Fedeli SL, Catalano G. Octreotide versus loperamide in the treatment of fluorouracil-induced diarrhoea: a randomized trial. J Clin Oncol. 1993;11:148–151.
89. Barbounis V, Koumakis G, Vassilomanalakis M, Demiri M, Efremidis AP. Control of irinotecan-induced diarrhoea by octreotide after loperamide failure. Suppl Care Cancer. 2001;9:258–60.
90. Meropol NJ, Blumenson LE, Creaven PJ. Octreotide does not prevent diarrhoea in patients treated with weekly 5-fluorouracil plus high-dose leucovorin. Am J Clin Oncol. 1998;2:135–8.
91. Simon DM, Cello JP, Valenzuela J et al. Multicenter trial of octreotide in patients with refractory acquired immunodeficiency syndrome-associated diarrhoea. Gastroentrology. 1995;108:1753–60.
92. van der Hulst RR, van Kreel BK, von Meyenfeldt MF et al. Glutamine and the preservation of gut integrity. Lancet. 1993;341:1363–5.
93. Tremel H, Kienle B, Weilemann LS, Stehle P, Furst P. Glutamine dipeptide-supplemented parenteral nutrition maintains intestinal function in the critically ill. Gastroenterology. 1994;107:1595–601.
94. Fox AD, Kripke SA, De Paula J, Berman JM, Settle RG, Rombeau JL. Effect of a glutamine-supplemented enteral diet on methotrexate-induced enterocolitis. J Parent Ent Nutr. 1988;12:325–31.
95. Rombeau JL. A review of the effects of glutamine-enriched diets on experimentally induced enterocolitis. J Parent Ent Nutr. 1990;14(Suppl.):100–5S.
96. Decker-Baumann C, Buhl K, Frohmüller S, Herbay A v, Dueck M, Schlag PM. Reduction of chemotherapy-induced side-effects by parenteral glutamine supplementation in patients with colorectal cancer. Eur J Cancer. 1999;35:202–7.
97. Savarese D, Al-Zoubi A, Boucher J. Glutamine for irinotecan diarrhoea. J Clin Oncol. 2000;18:450.
98. Ikegami T, Ha L, Arimori K et al. Intestinal alkalization as a possible preventive mechanism in irinotecan (CPT-11)-induced diarrhoea. Cancer Res. 2002;62:179–87.
99. Gandia D, Abigerges D, Armand JP et al. CPT-11-induced cholinergic effects in cancer patients. J Clin Oncol. 1993;11:196–7.
100. Govindarajan R, Heaton KM, Broadwater R, Zeitlin A, Lang NP, Hauer-Jensen M. Effect of thalidomide on gastrointestinal toxic effects of irinotecan. Lancet. 2000;356:566.
101. Lenfers BH, Loeffler TM, Droege CM, Hausamen TU. Substantial activity of budenoside in patients with irinotecan (CPT-11) and 5-flourouacil induced diarrhoea and failure of loperamide treatment. Ann Oncol. 1999;10:1251–53.
102. Wolf H. Preclinical and clinical pharmacology of the 5-HT3 receptor antagonists. Scand J Rheumatol. 2000;113:37–45.
103. Bailey LD Jr, Stewart WR Jr, McCallum RW. New directions in the irritable bowel syndrome. Gastroenterol Clin N Am. 1991;20:335–49.
104. Steadman CJ, Talley NJ, Phillips SF, Zinsmeister AR. Selective 5-hydroxytryptamine type 3 receptor antagonism with ondansetron as treatment for diarrhoea-predominant irritable bowel syndrome: a pilot study. Mayo Clin Proc. 1992;67:732–8.
105. Nightingale JM, Walker ER, Burnham WR, Farthing MJ, Lennard-Jones JE. Short bowel syndrome. Digestion. 1990;45(Suppl.):77–83.
106. Mennie AT, Dalley VM, Dinneen LC, Collier HO. Treatment of radiation-induced gastrointestinal distress with acetylsalicylate. Lancet. 1975;2:942–3.
107. Wadler S, Haynes H, Wiernik PH. Phase I trial of the somatostatin analog octreotide acetate in the treatment of fluoropyrimidine-induced diarrhoea. J Clin Oncol. 1995;13:222–6.
108. US Department of Health and Human Services, National Institutes of Health, National Cancer Institute. Investigator's Handbook: a manual for participants in clinical trials of investigational agents sponsored by DCTD, NCI. Bethesda, MD: National Cancer Institute, 1993.

15
Disturbances of pancreatic exocrine function, pancreatitis

J. MÖSSNER

DISTURBANCES OF PANCREATIC EXOCRINE FUNCTION

Chemotherapy usually does not induce exocrine pancreatic insufficiency that needs enzyme substitution. In patients with diabetic predisposition treatment with glucocorticosteroids may induce overt insulin-dependent diabetes.

ACUTE PANCREATITIS

Among the causes leading to acute pancreatitis drugs account for about 2%. These drugs include medications used in tumour therapy. Drug-induced pancreatitis may be separated into several groups (Table 1)[1–5]:

1. definite association (numerous case reports, relapse of pancreatitis after rechallenge);
2. probable association;
3. possible but questionable association.

Some drugs are discussed controversially in the literature regarding the group to which they belong[1–5].

There are more potential causes for acute pancreatitis during antineoplastic tumour therapy:

1. iatrogenic causes due to diagnostic or therapeutic procedures such as ERCP, abdominal surgery, chemoembolization of liver arteries;
2. additional drugs such as antibiotics, analgesics, immunosuppressive drugs;
3. infections such as Cytomegalovirus infection in patients with AIDS;
4. metastases of the pancreas.

Pancreatitis due to chemotherapy is a relatively rare event; however, severe and lethal courses are possible. One should thus consider this complication,

Table 1 Drug-induced pancreatitis (antineoplastic chemotherapeutic agents in bold)

Definite association	*Probable association*	*Possible but questionable association*
ACE inhibitors	Anticholinesterases	Acetaminophen
5-Aminosalicyclic acid	Antituberculous agents: isoniazid, rifampicin	Allopurinol
L-Asparaginase: <2%, pegaspargase: <18% ?	Biguanides	Amphotericin B
Azathioprine, 6-mercaptopurine	Clozapine	Antiviral agents used in HIV
Oestrogens	Contrast media in ERCP	Chlorthalidone
Lipid-lowering drugs: bezafibrate, simvastatin	**Glucocorticosteroids**	Clonidine
Loop diuretics: furosemide, ethacrynic acid	H_2-blocking agents: cimetidine	Codeine
Methimazole	Calcium 2′3′-dideoxyinosine/danosin	**Combination chemotherapy: e.g. busulfan/cyclophosphamide/ etoposide**
Methyldopa	Metronidazole	Cyclosporin
NSAR: sulindac	Methyldopa	**Cytarabine**
Sulphonamides	Pentamidine	Danazol (anabolic steroid)
Tetracyclines, minocycline (in CF)	**Cisplatinum**	Diphenhydramine
Thiazides: chlorothiazide, hydrochlorodiazide	Sulphasalazine	Erythromycin, roxythromycin
Valproic acid	Sodium stibogluconate, further pentavalent antimonial agents (used in treatment of leishmaniasis)	Estramustine phosphate
Vinca alkaloids	Zalcitabine	Griseofulvines; interferons; NSAR: ketoprofen, piroxicam; lithium; metolazone; nitrofurantoin; octreotide; paracetamol; **paclitaxel;** paromomycin (treatment of cryptosporidiosis in AIDS); phenformin; polyethylene glycol; procainamide; **retinoids, e.g. bexarotene**, isotretinoin used in treatment of acne; serotonin type 3 antagonists; sulphonamides, sulphamethoxazole-trimethoprim; **tamoxifen**; ticlopin; warfarin

especially since the typical symptoms may be obscured by other tumour symptoms or symptoms due to therapy.

Due to the numerous drugs applied during tumour therapy, identification of the responsible drug may be difficult; thus the decision as to which drug should be omitted may be a real challenge.

Pathomechanism

Hypertriglyceridaemia is a well-known cause of acute pancreatitis. In primary disturbances of lipid metabolism additional presence of the so-called four D's, i.e. drugs, diseases, diet (alcohol!), and disorder of metabolism, may lead to aggravation of hyperlipidaemia. Among those drugs are liposomal amphotericin B, ß-blockers, glucocorticosteroids, oestrogens, retinoids, tamoxifen, and thiazides.

Following allogenic bone marrow transplantation acute pancreatitis, often subclinical, is not so rare. Sludge in the common bile duct due to 'graft-versus-host' disease, Cytomegalovirus infection of the pancreas, toxic side-effects of immunosuppressive drugs such as cyclosporin, prednisone, etc., are considered as relevant factors in pathogenesis. Cases of acute pancreatitis are reported due to immunosuppressive therapy after kidney transplantation.

Pancreatitis due to liposomal amphotericin B, drug-induced hyperlipidaemia, liposomes by themselves or toxic effects may play a causative role.

Further potential pathomechanisms may include instant or prolonged immune reactions, elevation of pancreatic duct pressure due to osmotic effects, thrombosis of pancreatic arteries, obstructions of pancreatic ducts, metabolic and toxic effects.

Therapy

Usually immediate cessation of application of the responsible drug is mandatory. Rechallenge with the drug with an association with pancreatitis documented in the literature should be strictly avoided. Drug-induced pancreatitis may take a severe and lethal course.

CHRONIC PANCREATITIS

Chronic pancreatitis as consequence of a continuation of drug therapy is a rather rare event.

PANCREATIC CARCINOMA

Following polychemotherapy, e.g. leukaemia or lymphoma, or following long-term immunosuppressive therapy, e.g. after kidney transplantation or bone marrow transplantation, secondary neoplasias are possible. Pancreatic carcinoma may belong to these secondary tumours; however, this is very rare.

THERAPY WITH 5-FLUOROURACIL

In the Russian literature successful therapy of acute pancreatitis with 5-fluorouracil (5-FU) has been reported. Inhibition of protein synthesis has been claimed to be responsible for this beneficial effect; however, there are no placebo-controlled prospective double-blind studies that prove the findings of these case reports. We have shown, using the model of isolated rat pancreatic acini, that 5-FU has no effect on pancreatic enzyme secretion or on protein synthesis[6].

References

1. Andersen V, Sonne J, Andersen M. Spontaneous reports on drug-induced pancreatitis in Denmark from 1968 to 1999. Eur J Clin Pharmacol. 2001;57:517–21.
2. Frick TW, Speiser DE, Bimmler D, Largiader F. Drug-induced acute pancreatitis: further criticism. Dig Dis. 1993;11:113–32.
3. Nakashima Y, Howard JM. Drug-induced acute pancreatitis. Surg Gynecol Obstet. 1977;145:105–9.
4. Underwood TW, Frye CB. Drug-induced pancreatitis. Clin Pharm. 1993;12:440–8.
5. Wilmink T, Frick TW. Drug-induced pancreatitis. Drug Safety. 1996;14:406–23.
6. Bielecki K, Wiedmann M, Meyer F, Kimura W, Mössner J. Effect of 5-fluorouracil on secretion and synthesis of pancreatic digestive enzymes. Studies in isolated pancreatic acini and perfused pancreas derived from normal rats and from rats with acute necrotizing pancreatitis. Pancreas. 1994;9:518–25.

16 Chemotherapy and liver function

G. RAMADORI and T. ARMBRUST

THE LIVER IS THE CENTRAL ORGAN OF INTERMEDIATE METABOLISM, BUT CRUCIAL IN HOST DEFENCE

The liver hosts a variety of cell types. The parenchymal cells, the hepatocytes, comprise about 90% of the liver mass and about 60% of the total number of liver cells; they are responsible for the functions of the organ that are most prominent: organization and performance of intermediate metabolism, and metabolic detoxification and excretion of waste products. This high biosynthetic activity is achieved by a high ribosomal content of hepatocytes, and cellular DNA replication (DNA endoreplication) resulting in polyploidy or even in several nuclei per cell. In case of any abnormalities due to hepatocellular damage on one hand, or a high demand for hepatocellular biosynthesis on the other hand, this high-powered engine may get into trouble. Details on this problem in the context of systemic cytotoxic chemotherapy will be discussed below.

As well as the well-known functions of the liver regarding intermediate metabolism and detoxification, there is another, not so prominent, but in the long run probably equally relevant function, the clearance function[1]. For a good reason about 80% of the body's fixed tissue macrophages reside within the liver. They have been known as Kupffer cells[2] and are in direct contact with the blood streaming back from the gut. This blood may be heavily loaded with toxic agents (lipopolysaccharide) or infectious agents (bacteria, viruses), cellular debris, undigested biomaterial or any other compounds that are not supposed to enter the blood, but do so due to the high permissiveness of the gut epithelial lining. Scavenging of all this material is achieved in the liver[1] by Kupffer cell and sinusoidal endothelial cell endocytosis[3]. Macro- and micropinocytosis of small particulate and fluid matter by sinusoidal endothelial cells, and phagocytosis of particulate material and of cells by Kupffer cells – either by unspecific binding and uptake or by receptor-mediated uptake – represent the basic principles of hepatic clearance. Moreover, humoral factors that are part of the innate immune system synthesized and released by hepatic cells may ease hepatic clearance.

A paradigm of an innate immunity is given by the elaborate complement system[4,5]. Initialized by immunocomplexes (e.g. immunoglobulins bound to bacteria or viruses) or by unspecific mechanisms, a cascade of proteins is activated, resulting in lysis of microorganisms, or in surface-binding and endocytosis by phagocytes. Many of these complement proteins are synthesized by hepatocytes, Kupffer cells[6,7], and other non-parenchymal liver cells[8]. Non-complement factors may facilitate recognition of foreign matter by phagocytic cells and thus ease endocytosis. This procedure is referred to as opsonization. Plasma fibronectin, a multifunctional glycoprotein, has such an opsonic activity, and is abundantly secreted by hepatocytes[9]. Changes in the function of the liver immune cells have been reported after cytotoxic chemotherapy, and will be discussed below.

BASIC PRINCIPLES OF CYTOTOXIC CHEMOTHERAPY

Chemotherapy as the main non-surgical remedy of cancer treatment is generally based on the cytotoxic effect of natural or synthetic agents taking advantage of a higher vulnerability of cancer cells as compared to normal cells. However, normal cells may also be affected by cytotoxic chemotherapy[10]. Susceptibility to chemotherapy is linked to the proliferative rate of a cell population as seen in bone marrow cells or mucosal cells with high replication rates. The cytotoxic effect of chemotherapy may be permitted via different targets within cells. Inhibition of DNA replication and transcription via interference of cancer drugs, either with the DNA strand, enzymes involved in DNA metabolism, or DNA substrates, may rank as the most important principle of cancer treatment directly inhibiting cell proliferation. Moreover, inhibition of RNA and protein synthesis constitute an attempt to inhibit cancer cell growth.

THE LIVER IS A TARGET OF, AND SUFFERING FROM, CYTOTOXIC CHEMOTHERAPY

As stated above, cancer cells as well as normal cells are affected by chemotherapeutics. Replication of hepatocytes is low in normal liver, but may reach a dramatic level during liver regeneration after massive hepatocellular death or partial hepatectomy. However, during cytotoxic chemotherapy that is performed only in patients with normal or near-normal liver function, inhibition of hepatocellular replication is thus not of primary importance. Nevertheless, systemic application of chemotherapeutics affecting DNA, RNA, or protein synthesis affects hepatocellular function in several ways.

A main side-effect of chemotherapy, nausea and vomiting, causes fasting of patients after therapy. Reduced uptake of nutrients has been shown to induce a shrinkage of the liver that may achieve a reduction in liver cell mass of almost 50% under total starvation. Normal food uptake after fasting has been shown to induce high DNA synthesis in hepatocytes without cellular replication (DNA endoreplication) resulting in polyploidy and the presence of several nuclei in some hepatocytes. However, even without a period of fasting, high-powered hepatocytes demanding normal DNA, RNA and protein synthesis are affected by reduced DNA synthesis in hepatocytes[11].

IMPACT OF CYTOTOXIC CHEMOTHERAPY ON LIVER FUNCTION: HEPATOCELLULAR DYSFUNCTION AND CLINICAL IMPLICATIONS

Up to 85% of patients receiving chemotherapy develop liver steatosis, indicating disturbed lipid metabolism via altered lipoprotein synthesis by hepatocytes and finally resulting in hepatocellular lipid accumulation. The latter induces higher vulnerability of hepatocytes that may, in particular during repeated chemotherapy, induce irreversible hepatocellular damage. Elevation of serum aminotransferases may thus be explained, and represents a frequent event during or after cytotoxic chemotherapy. The hepatocellular sensibility to cytotoxic chemotherapy depends on the particular chemotherapeutic used, giving rise to a classification of agents with high or low potential hepatotoxicity (Table 1). Moreover, it is a characteristic for a single chemotherapeutic to exert its hepatotoxic potential at low or only at high dosages[4,12]. In some cases prolonged hepatotoxicity may be observed after a single application, e.g. after asparaginase treatment[13]. After repeated methotrexate treatments the occurrence of liver cirrhosis has been reported[14,15].

The metabolization and detoxification of many chemotherapeutics in the liver[16] depends on the activity of a particular enzyme pathway that may be altered by hepatocellular dysfunction induced by itself. Moreover, genetic variations[17,18] or inhibition of degrading enzymes by non-cytotoxic drugs may delay hepatic metabolization of the cytotoxic agent, thus increasing its toxicity. A contrary effect may be observed if the cytotoxic agent is in need of activation by a hepatic enzyme (prodrugs)[19], or if a non-cytotoxic drug increases the expression of a hepatic enzyme (Table 2).

Impaired detoxification may be accompanied by disturbed biliary excretion of hepatocytes due to chemotherapy-induced slow-down of hepatocellular metabolism inducing elevation of serum parameters of cholestasis (Table 3).

Table 1 Hepatotoxicity of cytotoxic chemotherapeutics

High potential hepatotoxicity
Asparaginase, methotrexate, cytarabine, streptozocin
High potential hepatotoxicity if given in high dosages
Busulfan, dactinomycin, carmustin, mitomycin, cyclophosphamide, methotrexate, cytarabin, diaziquone
Irreversible hepatotoxicity (rare)
Azathioprine, dacarbazin, busulfan, methotrexate, carmustine, mitomycin, cytarabin
Low potential hepatotoxicity
Azathioprin, 6-mercaptopurine, dacarbazin, pentostatin, hydroxyurea, 6-thioguanine, vincristine

Table 2 Liver chemotherapeutics – metabolizing enzymes and interaction with drugs

Drug-metabolizing enzymes		*Interaction*
Cytochrome P450		
CYP2B6	Cyclophosphamide	
CYP2C8	Paclitaxel	
CYP3A4	Etoposide	Ketoconazole (d)
	Vinca alkaloids	Erythromycin (d)
	Ifosfamide	Grapefruit juice (d)
	Docetaxel	Corticosteroids (u)
	Irinotecan	Phenytoin (u)
Ketoreductase	Anthracyclins	
Carboxylesterases	Irinotecan	
Dihydropyrimidine dehydrogenase	5-Fluorouracil	

(d), down-regulation of the enzyme by the agent; (u), up-regulation.

Table 3 Hepatic side-effects of chemotherapeutics

Steatosis hepatitis
All chemotherapeutics
Elevation of aminotransferases
Cytarabin
Nitrosourea
Liver cirrhosis
Methotrexate
Cholestasis, hepatocellular necrosis
6-Mercaptopurine
Mithramycin
Cholecystitis, cholangitis
FUDR
Veno-occlusive disease
Busulfan, nitrosourea, mitomycin C

IMPAIRMENT OF LIVER FUNCTION DURING CYTOTOXIC CHEMOTHERAPY: IMPACT ON CLEARANCE FUNCTION

As stated above, the liver is the home of 80% of all fixed tissue macrophages of the body. It must be assumed that this accumulation of mononuclear phagocytes in the liver reflects a high demand for clearance in this particular organ primarily conducted by Kupffer cells (Table 4). Interestingly, the turnover of Kupffer cells has been debated for decades, and there is no final concordance as to what extent Kupffer cells are self-replicative or replaced by immigrating blood monocytes. However, Kupffer cells have a long life-span, in the range of several months. The mitotic index is quite low, and increasing evidence has accumulated showing that

Kupffer cells primarily derive from bone marrow cells[20]. Accordingly, a sizeable population of transient monocytes has been reported in normal liver[21]. On the other hand, a large influx of blood monocytes is observed in the diseased liver[22].

After chemotherapy with suppression of bone marrow cell replication the supply of Kupffer cell precursor cells is disturbed. Because gut lining epithelial cell replication is also suppressed, a subsequently increased permeability of the gut gives rise to a greatly increased hepatic onflow of toxic and infectious agents demanding a faster turnover of hepatic macrophages. This divergency may result in an increased risk of infections (Figure 1).

It has also been shown that cytotoxic chemotherapy impairs the phagocytotic activity of Kupffer cells. After treatment of Kupffer cells with mitomycin-c

Table 4 Kupffer cell clearance

Foreign particulate material
Microorganisms
Endotoxin
Immune complexes
Cellular debris and enzymes
Erythrocytes
Apoptotic granulocytes
Tumour cells
Modified LDLs
Portal antigens

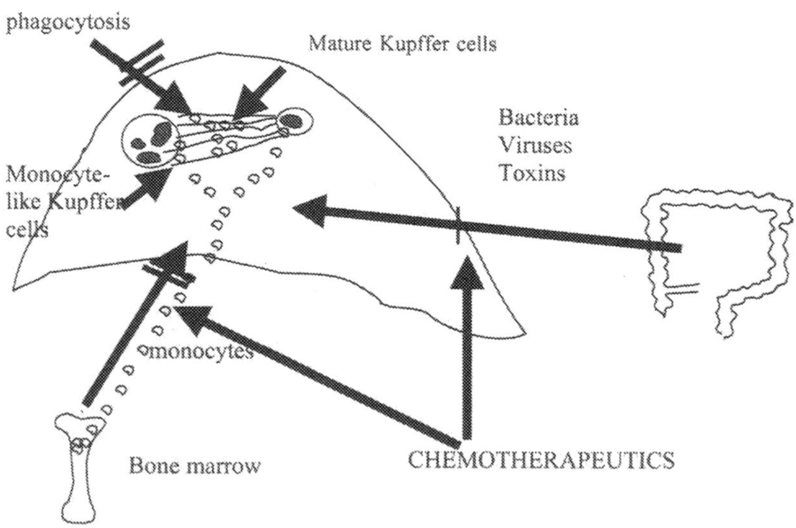

Figure 1 Effect of chemotherapeutics on liver clearance function. Reduced replacement of Kupffer cells by suppression of bone marrow supply of blood monocytes. Reduced phagocytotic activity of Kupffer cells. Increased permeability of intestinal mucosa

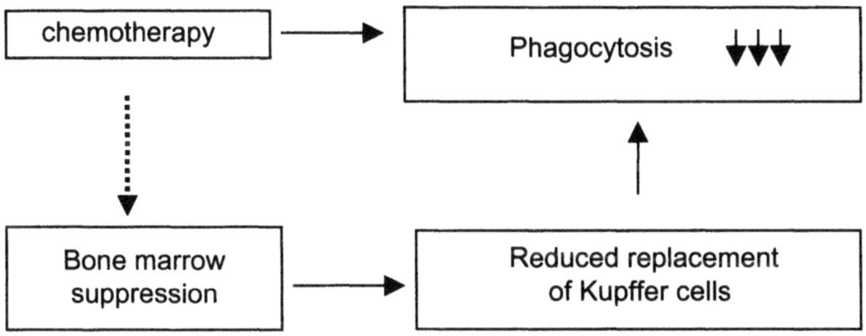

Figure 2 Kupffer cell clearance: impairment by chemotherapeutics

Table 5 Effects of cytotoxic chemotherapy on liver clearance function

First line of defence	Central organ of innate immunity
↓	↓
Synthesis of humoral factors	Main organ of RES
↓ reduced synthesis	↓
Hepatocytes: complement factors	Reduced phagocytosis
haemoxygenase-1 clotting factors fibronectin	↓ Infections
Kupffer cells: complement factors cytokines oxygen radicals haemoxygenase-1 IGF-BP-3	

phagocytosis was reduced by up to 75% as compared to control cultures. Reduced phagocytotic activity was observed for up to 4 weeks after treatment[23] (Figure 2). Reduced synthesis of humoral factors of host defence by hepatocytes may also be critical in the development of infections after cytotoxic chemotherapy (Table 5).

VENO-OCCLUSIVE DISEASE OF THE LIVER

Bone marrow transplantation in conjunction with chemotherapy is a major risk factor for development of veno-occlusive disease (VOD) of the liver[24,25] (Table 6). The clinical hallmarks of the onset of this disease are sudden weight gain, hepatomegaly and jaundice accompanied by a high elevation of aminotransferases and hepatic encephalopathy. The basic pathophysiological mechanism of induction of VOD of the liver is presumed to be injury to the endothelial cells of central veins and sublobular liver veins[26]. A subsequent clotting activation

Table 6 Veno-occlusive disease of the liver

Classical triad
Rapid weight gain
Hepatomegaly
Jaundice
Pathophysiological events
Clotting activation
Pericentral hepatocellular necrosis
Narrowing of central veins
Thrombosis of central veins
Thrombosis of liver veins
Therapeutic options
Fibrinolysis
TIPS
Liver transplantation

results in occlusion of central veins, sublobular veins and, in the worst case, of liver veins. Fibrinolysis may have a positive effect on the outcome of this disease, and single cases of an emergency implantation of a transjugular portosystemic shunt (TIPS) have been reported[27]. However, the final option in preventing a fatal outcome is liver transplantation[28,29].

References

1. Toth CA, Thomas P. Liver endocytosis and Kupffer cells. Hepatology. 1992;16:255–66.
2. Jones EA, Kupffer cells. In: Arias JM, Popper H, Schachter D, Shafritz DA, editors. The Liver: Biology and Pathobiology. New York: Raven Press, 1988:683–704.
3. Rieder H, Meyer zum Buschenfelde KH, Ramadori G. Functional spectrum of sinusoidal endothelial liver cells. Filtration, endocytosis, synthetic capacities and intercellular communication. J Hepatol. 1992;15:237–50.
4. Morgan BP. The complement system: an overview. Methods Mol Biol. 2000;150:1–13.
5. Song WC, Sarrias MR, Lambris JD. Complement and innate immunity. Immunopharmacology. 2000;49:187–98.
6. Armbrust T et al. C1Q synthesis by tissue mononuclear phagocytes from normal and from damaged rat liver: up-regulation by dexamethasone, down-regulation by interferon gamma, and lipopolysaccharide. Hepatology. 1997;26:98–106.
7. Armbrust T et al. C1 esterase inhibitor gene expression in rat Kupffer cells, peritoneal macrophages and blood monocytes: modulation by interferon gamma. J Exp Med. 1993; 178:373–80.
8. Schwogler S et al. Fat-storing cells of the rat liver synthesize and secrete C1-esterase inhibitor; modulation by cytokines. Hepatology. 1992;16:794–802.
9. Hynes R. Molecular biology of fibronectin. Annu Rev Cell Biol. 1985;1:67–90.
10. Debatin KM. Cytotoxic drugs, programmed cell death, and the immune system: defining new roles in an old play. J Natl Cancer Inst. 1997;89:750–1.
11. Skullman S, Ihse I, Larsson J. Influence of malnutrition on regeneration and composition of the liver in rats. Acta Chir Scand. 1990;156:717–22.
12. Moertel CG et al. Hepatic toxicity associated with fluorouracil plus levamisole adjuvant therapy. J Clin Oncol. 1993;11:2386–90.
13. Jenkins R, Perlin E. Severe hepatotoxicity from *Escherichia coli* L-asparaginase. J Natl Med Assoc. 1987;79:775–9.
14. Furst DE. Methotrexate: new mechanisms and old toxicities. Agents Actions Suppl. 1993; 44:131–7.
15. West SG. Methotrexate hepatotoxicity. Rheum Dis Clin N Am. 1997;23:883–915.
16. Sitar DS. Human drug metabolism *in vivo*. Pharmacol Ther. 1989;43:363–75.

17. Taningher M et al. Drug metabolism polymorphisms as modulators of cancer susceptibility. Mutat Res. 1999;436:227–61.
18. Diasio RB, Beavers TL, Carpenter JT. Familial deficiency of dihydropyrimidine dehydrogenase. Biochemical basis for familial pyrimidinemia and severe 5-fluorouracil-induced toxicity. J Clin Invest. 1988;81:47–51.
19. Ferguson MJ, Ahmed FY, Cassidy J. The role of pro-drug therapy in the treatment of cancer. Drug Resist Update. 2001;4:225–32.
20. Wake K et al. Cell biology and kinetics of Kupffer cells in the liver. Int Rev Cytol. 1989; 118:173–229.
21. Armbrust T, Ramadori G. Functional characterization of two different Kupffer cell populations of normal rat liver. J Hepatol. 1996;25:518–28.
22. Armbrust T, Ramadori G. Mononuclear phagocytes of acutely injured rat liver abundantly synthesize and secrete fibronectin in contrast to Kupffer cells of normal liver. Biochem Biophys Res Commun. 1995;213:752–8.
23. Bodenheimer H Jr, Charland C, Leith J. Alteration of rat Kupffer cell function following mitomycin-C administration. J Leukoc Biol. 1988;43:265–70.
24. Bearman SI. Veno-occlusive disease of the liver. Curr Opin Oncol. 2000;12:103–9.
25. Baron F, Deprez M, Beguin Y. The veno-occlusive disease of the liver. Haematologica. 1997;82: 718–25.
26. DeLeve LD, Shulman HM, McDonald GB. Toxic injury to hepatic sinusoids: sinusoidal obstruction syndrome (veno-occlusive disease). Semin Liver Dis. 2002;22:27–42.
27. de la Rubia J et al. Successful treatment of hepatic veno-occlusive disease in a peripheral blood progenitor cell transplant patient with a transjugular intrahepatic portosystemic stent-shunt (TIPS). Haematologica. 1996;81:536–9.
28. Schlitt HJ et al. Allogeneic liver transplantation for hepatic veno-occlusive disease after bone marrow transplantation – clinical and immunological considerations. Bone Marrow Transplant. 1995;16:473–8.
29. Norris S et al. Orthotopic liver transplantation for veno-occlusive disease complicating autologous bone marrow transplantation. Transplantation. 1997;63:1521–4.

Section V
Perspectives, alternatives

17
Specific immunotherapy, angiogenesis inhibitors, gene therapy and other approaches: do we still need chemotherapy?

D. JÄGER

INTRODUCTION

Chemotherapy is still one of the standard treatment modalities for most malignancies. Over recent years different approaches have been developed in order to selectively target tumour cells without harming normal tissues. This chapter addresses some of the newer treatment approaches that either recently became available, or that are currently being evaluated in different cancer treatment regimens.

SPECIFIC IMMUNOTHERAPY

Active specific immunotherapy uses the host's immune system to elicit a cellular immune response ($CD4^+$ or $CD8^+$ T cells) against specific tumour antigens. Several categories of tumour antigens have been identified to date[1], namely: (1) 'cancer-testis' antigens, which are expressed in cancers of different histological type and normal testicular tissue, or germal cells, but not in any other normal tissue; (2) differentiation antigens are expressed in a differentiated normal tissue and its malignant counterpart (i.e. melanocyte and melanoma, or breast tissue and breast cancer); (3) antigens that are overexpressed in tumour tissue; (4) mutated antigens; (5) (retro)viral antigens; (6) splice-variant antigens. The 'ideal' target antigen for active immunotherapy should be highly and homogeneously expressed in a variety of different tumours; it should be highly immunogenic; finally there should be no or low expression in normal tissues.

Active immunotherapy can be performed as peptide immunization (peptides derived from the tumour antigen)[2,3]. Alternatively the whole protein can be used to immunize patients, as well as naked DNA, RNA or virus constructs encoding the tumour antigen. All these approaches have been shown to be effective in eliciting an antigen-specific $CD4^+$ or $CD8^+$ T cell response. NY-ESO-1, a cancer-testis antigen originally identified in oesophageal cancer[4], is thought to be the most immunogenic cancer antigen for tumour vaccination to date. Clinical studies using NY-ESO-1 derived peptides, protein, or viral constructs encoding the full-length protein, have been shown to be effective in eliciting an antigen-specific $CD8^+$ T cell response[3,5,6]. The T cell response is reflected by the intensity of the DTH reaction, and can be detected by ELISPOT assays or tetramer analysis. No side-effects have been observed to date, with some patients achieving clinical remissions[3].

The optimal route of vaccination (intradermal, intranodal, etc.) and the optimal adjuvant (GM-CSF, IL-12, IL-2, CpG, etc.) is currently unknown and under investigation. Future vaccine trials will show if polyvalent vaccines targeting different antigens simultaneously result in improved clinical outcome.

PASSIVE IMMUNOTHERAPY

This treatment modality uses monoclonal antibodies directed against cell surface antigens highly expressed on tumour cells. Passive immunotherapy can be performed in combination with chemotherapy, and results from some larger clinical trials show the efficacy of this combined treatment modality, i.e. monoclonal antibody targeting CD20 on B cells and Her2/neu on breast cancer cells combined with chemotherapy are already part of standard treatment protocols. Other cell surface antigens, such as CD33 on myeloid cells, A33 on colon cancer[7], are currently being evaluated for clinical use.

A different form of passive immunotherapy is the adoptive transfer of T cells. For this approach *ex-vivo* stimulated $CD8^+$ T cells are expanded in culture and reinfused to the cancer patient. The data from several early clinical trials show excellent tolerability and some remissions in individual patients.

INHIBITORS OF CELL PROLIFERATION AND ANGIOGENESIS

The identification and understanding of cell signalling pathways involved in cell cycle regulation, proliferation, adhesion, and apoptosis have opened up an array of new targets for intervention in cancer therapy. Today, with the development of specific tyrosine kinase inhibitors (TKI), specific signalling pathways in cancer cells may be blocked with induction of cell cycle arrest and/or apoptosis. There is a whole array of new TKI in early clinical evaluation. STI571 (Imatinib, Gleevec) is a TKI that specifically blocks the bcr-abl TKI in chronic myelogenic leukaemia, but also platelet-derived growth factor (PDGF), stem cell factor (SCF), and c-kit. STI571 has shown impressive clinical results in CML, and is also becoming a treatment option in c-kit positive tumours such as GIST[8].

Another TKI that blocks signalling pathways mediated by the epidermal growth factor receptor (EGFR) has shown some promising clinical results. EGFR is highly expressed on most epithelial tumour cells but also in normal epithelial and mesenchymal cells. ZD1839 (iressa) has a strong anti-angiogenesis activity; it reduces cell motility and adhesion, and promotes apoptosis[9]. ZD1839 is well tolerated with moderate toxicity; it is available as an oral medication. Several clinical trials with ZD1839 in combination with chemotherapy are currently under way. Recently it was approved in Japan for the treatment of NSCLC. Several monoclonal antibodies targeting EGFR and variant EGFR/EGFR mutations are currently in clinical trials. Due to the cancer-specific expression patterns of ΔEGFR and mutated EGFR, a more selective killing of cancer cells may be achieved when targeting these molecules.

INDUCTION OF TUMOUR CELL DIFFERENTIATION

Tumour cells show a different gene expression profile than do normal tissue cells. By activating silenced genes in tumour cells those undifferentiated cells can be transformed into more differentiated cells with less proliferative activity. Valproic acid, a drug that has been widely used in the treatment of epilepsy, is an inhibitor of histone deacetylase, which represents one mechanism of transcriptional regulation. It could be shown *in vitro* that myeloid blast cells in AML can be transformed into more differentiated myeloid cells by inhibiting histone deacetylase with valproic acid[10,11]. To evaluate the potential of valproic acid in cancer therapy, clinical phase I/II trials have been started.

GENE THERAPY

Tumour cells frequently acquire mutations, and some of the mutated genes are characteristic for the malignant disease, e.g. k-ras mutations in pancreatic cancer, or p53 mutations in NSCLC. Approaches to restore the original function of the mutated gene in a given tumour have so far failed to produce any beneficial results with respect to clinical outcome. Genetically engineered tumour cells such as GM-CSF transfected irradiated melanoma cells have been used to induce strong immune responses in active immunotherapy[12]. However, these approaches are technically quite involved and cumbersome, and although well tolerated, have not resulted in convincing remissions in cancer patients.

SUMMARY

The combination of chemotherapy with monoclonal antibodies is already an established treatment modality in B-cell neoplasias and Her2/neu$^+$ breast cancer. The development of specific tyrosine kinase inhibitors has produced promising results in some cancer types; the most prominent example is STI571 (Gleevec) in the treatment of CML. Active immunotherapy is an intriguing treatment modality in cancer, with promising results in multiple phase I/II trials. A thorough understanding of pathological molecular pathways in tumour cells will suggest more specific targets for new treatments in a variety of different malignant diseases. At this time, however, chemotherapy still remains an indispensable cornerstone in the management of most cancers.

References

1. Old LJ, Chen YT. New paths in human cancer serology. J Exp Med. 1998;187:1163–7.
2. Jaeger E, Bernhard H, Romero P et al. Generation of cytotoxic T-cell responses with synthetic melanoma-associated peptides *in vivo*: implications for tumor vaccines with melanoma-associated antigens. Int J Cancer. 1996;66:162–9.
3. Jager E, Chen YT, Drijfhout JW et al. Simultaneous humoral and cellular immune response against cancer-testis antigen NY-ESO-1: definition of human histocompatibility leukocyte antigen (HLA)-A2-binding peptide epitopes. J Exp Med. 1998;187:265–70.
4. Chen YT, Scanlan MJ, Sahin U et al. A testicular antigen aberrantly expressed in human cancers detected by autologous antibody screening. Proc Natl Acad Sci USA. 1997;94:1914–18.
5. Jager E, Gnjatic S, Nagata Y et al. Induction of primary NY-ESO-1 immunity: $CD8^+$ T lymphocyte and antibody responses in peptide-vaccinated patients with NY-ESO-1+ cancers. Proc Natl Acad Sci USA. 2000;97:12198–203.
6. Jager E, Nagata Y, Gnjatic S et al. Monitoring CD8 T cell responses to NY-ESO-1: correlation of humoral and cellular immune responses. Proc Natl Acad Sci USA. 2000;97:4760–5.
7. Welt S, Divgi CR, Real FX et al. Quantitative analysis of antibody localization in human metastatic colon cancer: a phase I study of monoclonal antibody A33. J Clin Oncol. 1990; 8:1894–906.
8. Attoub S, Rivat C, Rodrigues S et al. The c-kit tyrosine kinase inhibitor STI571 for colorectal cancer therapy. Cancer Res. 2002;62:4879–83.
9. Huang SM, Li J, Armstrong EA, Harari PM. Modulation of radiation response and tumor-induced angiogenesis after epidermal growth factor receptor inhibition by ZD1839 (Iressa). Cancer Res. 2002;62:4300–6.
10. Blaheta RA, Cinatl J Jr. Anti-tumor mechanisms of valproate: a novel role for an old drug. Med Res Rev. 2002;22:492–511.
11. Gottlicher M, Minucci S, Zhu P et al. Valproic acid defines a novel class of HDAC inhibitors inducing differentiation of transformed cells. EMBO J. 2001;20:6969–78.
12. Leong SP, Enders-Zohr P, Zhou YM et al. Recombinant human granulocyte macrophage–colony stimulating factor (rhGM–CSF) and autologous melanoma vaccine mediate tumor regression in patients with metastatic melanoma. J Immunother. 1999;22:166–74.

Index

INDEX